THE CONSTANCE FISHER TRAGEDY

Bob Briggs

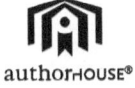

authorHOUSE®

AuthorHouse™
1663 Liberty Drive
Bloomington, IN 47403
www.authorhouse.com
Phone: 1-800-839-8640

First published by AuthorHouse 6/30/2011

ISBN: 978-1-4567-5645-1 (dj)
ISBN: 978-1-4567-5646-8 (e)
ISBN: 978-1-4567-5647-5 (sc)

Library of Congress Control Number: 2011908024

Printed in the United States of America

TABLE OF CONTENTS

ACKNOWLEDGMENTS

The writer would like to thank the following for their efforts in completing this manuscript:

Dr. Ulrich Jacobsohn for lending his expertise and support, a true pleasure to work with such a fine gentleman.

Michael Shepherd for helping me craft the original idea.

Sam Shain and Laura Fellows for their editorial support.

And Louise Bowker for opening up to us the world of her sister.

INTRODUCTION

My sister Peggy was a beautiful lady, a happy mother, loving wife and a devout Catholic. She was happy with her life. She LOVED her husband and her children. They were the center of her world. The children were very smart, active, outgoing and happy. She was a great cook; she enjoyed reading, sewing knitting and other crafts. She and Carl had a nice country house with lots of land and a large garden with both vegetables and flowers. Carl had a good job at the railroad and the family had a comfortable income.

She was hospitalized in the week prior to the second tragic episode in her life; the drowning of her children. My friend Fran Roy was the nursing supervisor on Peggy's hospital floor. Fran cried as she told me that that as she helped Peg to get ready for her discharge, she was crying. She told Fran that she was afraid to go home. Her doctor's response was, Go home & take care of your family. You ll be fine. He knew her history, she was begging for help. The medical community let Peggy down. Had her doctor paid attention and taken care of her needs, this never would have happened.

The Andrea Yates tragedy should never have happened. Her case was alarmingly parallel to my sister's. Again, the medical community let her down when she asked for help.

Please be aware of any mother you know who may be suffering from depression. Offer to take children of young mothers for a time to allow her to rest physically and mentally from the difficult daily job of motherhood. It is my understanding that these mothers experiencing extreme hormonal depression won t usually ask for help.

It is my sincere hope that this book will reach out and educate doctors and layman alike to recognize women like Peggy so that this kind of tragedy can be stopped. If this book helps to prevent even one other woman from hurting her family, Bob Briggs will have succeeded in his endeavor.

I miss my sister and will never have the pleasure of loving my nieces and nephews.

Louise Marcoux Bowker

DEDICATION

To Constance Fisher with the prayer that her sufferings were not in vain...

Now I think I know, what you tried to say to me...
How you suffered for your sanity...
How you tried to set them free...
But they would not listen, they did not know how...
Perhaps they'll listen now...

Don McLean
From the song, "Vincent"

CHAPTER ONE

DISASTER

"A voice was heard in Ramah, weeping and great mourning, Rachel weeping for her children; and she refused to be comforted, because they were no more."

Jeremiah 31:15

Monday, March 8, 1954 5:30 a.m.

THE SUN ROSE SLOWLY on a cold, snowy, day as the city of Waterville, Maine began to stir to life. Carl Fisher was up early, making his breakfast, packing his lunch, and waiting for his three youngsters to arise from their slumber.

He looked out on the steps that led to the ground from his second story flat to see if they needed shoveling. He checked the driveway and his 1949 Ford to see if he could slide out in time and not be late for work.

The Fisher children arose in their usual fashion. Richard, aged six and in the first grade, was always up first. He looked forward to watching Howdy Doody on TV before hurrying off to catch the school bus.

The happy face of the clown Clarabelle got the day off to a happy start. Ventriloquist Buffalo Bob Smith pulled the strings on the freck-

1

led-faced red-haired puppet, Howdy Doody, to provide an hour of entertainment for the recently discovered young audience. The show would end with Howdy singing jingles for commercials like the one for Halo shampoo, also makers of Selsum shampoo. Howdy would wave and sign off with the admonition of "see you tomorrow!" But there would be no tomorrow for Richard Fisher.

Following Richard to the television set was his sleepy eyed brother Daniel, aged five and a half-day student at the Sacred Heart Catholic school. The baby, Deborah, just short of one year old, was still asleep in the crib beside her mother, but would join them shortly.

After serving the children breakfast, and sending young Richard off to school, Carl Fisher went to the master bedroom to talk to his wife before he left for his job at the Maine Central Railroad. Most of the past week he had taken off to be with her as he could see her mood sinking into depression once again.

He brought his wife a cup of coffee and asked if she felt well enough for him to leave.

"I feel fine, Carl," she said. "I had a good nights sleep for the first time in weeks. It's okay, the kids and I will be fine."

But Carl Fisher had his doubts and suspicions...

The happy world that the Fishers had built began to fall apart shortly after the birth of their third child, Deborah. Feeling depressed and run down, Mrs. Fisher made an appointment to see Dr. Richard Chasse, who had delivered the child the past March.

The routine post partum check-up revealed that Mrs. Fisher had hypo-chromic anemia. Untreated, the condition often led to clinical depression, and feelings of fatigue. Dr. Chasse treated her with a high iron diet, and weekly injections of folic acid and vitamin B-12. In a couple of weeks, her blood work was normal, and Constance Fisher was feeling like her old self again.

But by November of 1953, Constance's health had again taken a turn for the worse. It was shortly after she stopped breast- feeding Deborah, the only child she weaned.

Constance was now at a point where everything bothered her. The baby crying, the dog barking, and Carl having an occasional beer. She saw bills mounting and no way to pay them. Christmas was right around the corner and it would not be much of a Christmas at the Fisher house.

Usually bubbly and full of the holiday spirit, Constance was slipping into a deepening valley of depression. Crying spells were frequent and triggered for no apparent reason. A pervading gloom seemed to snatch all her joy of living.

And then, out of nowhere, she began to hear voices. They sounded like a man's voice. They seemed to be an external one, not the voice of her inner thought life. They were always accompanied by a presence. They offered a solution to all of her problems: suicide.

Around Christmas, Constance began to get other ideas. Ideas like it would be better for all concerned if she killed not just herself, but the entire family.

The ideas incubated over the next three months before they finally hatched. When thought turned to action, she almost strangled her baby Deborah to death with a scarf.

It was in early January of 1954. While Carl was at work and the other children asleep, she wrapped a nylon scarf around the neck of little Debbie and began to pull it tight. When Constance heard the baby shriek, she resisted the temptation and frantically called Carl who left work and immediately returned home.

Not knowing what else to do, he took her to see Dr. Chasse again. Embarrassed and confused, Constance walked up the two flights of stairs to Dr. Chasse's office, before turning around and running back to the car.

Carl, however, convinced her to keep a new appointment for the next day. Together they agreed that the situation was spiraling way out of control.

Chasse prescribed a sedative to help Constance sleep and Phenobarbital to be taken at intervals throughout the day to ease her anxiety. Little was made about the incident with Deborah.

His report dated January 21, 1954 read:

> *This time she came to my office with her husband complaining of being run down, nervous, having a poor appetite and worrying a great deal about paying her bills and similar household problems. Physical examination revealed no astounding abnormity,*

either emotionally or physically. She complained of insomnia and
a pent up feeling inside...

I prescribed a mild sedative (Phenobarbital) to be taken in
doses of one teaspoonful after meals and at bedtime. I re-assured
the patient that she would improve and I was pleased that she was
so encouraged. I told her that if any more trouble in this manner
developed we would have her see a specialist for "nervous diseases"
to which she agreed. (1)

Dr. Chasse encouraged Carl to move his family from their secluded two-room cabin on Snow Pond, an extremely small space for a family of five people and two pets.

Although the family enjoyed living on the water, it was fraught with hardships. The was no indoor plumbing, or running water. They got drinking and bathing water from a spring, but in the winter had to chop through 3 to 4 inches of ice to scoop water from the lake.

And after a recent fire scare, Carl switched from oil to coal which produced an undesirable gas that Dr. Chasse felt might be contributing to Mrs. Fisher's problems.

Dr. Chasse also insisted that they were missing important social aspects by being so secluded from family and friends.

Carl Fisher agreed, and moved his family into the top floor of a duplex on 31 High Street in Waterville which was in proximity to Constance's foster parents, Warren and Ursula Marcoux.

At first the move was greeted with success. The money earned from the sale of the cabin was enough to pay off their debts and give them a small cushion. Constance was within walking distance of her mother, who helped with the children and the chores and was a companion while Carl was at work.

Mrs. Marcoux and her daughters Bunny and Virginia would take Constance shopping to break up the monotony of the day, or if she began to feel depressed, could show up at a moment's notice. The Marcoux's also contributed by buying a washing machine, installing a telephone, and buying them the chief novelty of the day; a black-and-white television set.

An avid reader, Constance once again began to find consolation and inspiration in books and magazines. It appeared to all concerned that Constance was getting over the hump of the depression that had plagued her by varying degrees since last summer.

In a new environment and buoyed by medication, Constance appeared to have a new lease on life. She told Dr. Chasse at an appointment on February 4, 1954, that she was sleeping well, enjoying shopping with her mother, and wishing that she had moved away from the cottage long before. She told Dr. Chasse that she was very pleased that she was much better now and that she no longer had the urge to kill her children...

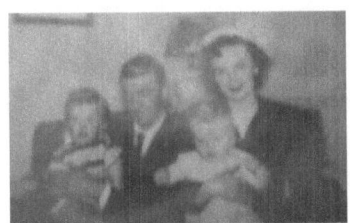

The Fisher family in 1950.
From right to left are: Richard, Carl, Daniel, and Constance.

Chasse gave her another physical examination and ordered a CBC which revealed that she was again anemic and advised her to begin an anti-emetic diet, with an oral iron supplement. He gave her intra-muscular injections of folic acid and B-12 and recommended that she see a specialist, Dr. Loring Pratt, for an inner ear infection that would not clear up.

After visiting Dr. Pratt's office, Constance left with an antibiotic and a prescription for a special shampoo for the psoriasis that Dr. Pratt believed was aggravating her ear condition. Dr. Pratt told her to be very careful of the shampoo, a Selsum product, as it contained a very poisonous ingredient.

"Please, keep it out of the reach of the children," he warned. And be sure to clean yourself thoroughly, even under your fingernails."

But the respite from her illness was once again short-lived. Despite the efforts of the doctors, Carl, who had now taken on a second job to pay for medical costs, and the support of her family, Constance once again lapsed into the black hole of depression.

Afraid for herself, her family, and what the future might bring, Constance Fisher was contemplating suicide again. On the night of February 11, shortly after supper, she swallowed the remainder of the bottle of Phenobarbital.

When Carl went to bed, he found his wife in a near comatose condition. He immediately phoned Dr. Sam Fisher who hurriedly came to the apartment and gave Constance an antidote for the drug turned poison. In the morning, Carl contacted Dr. Chasse.

Dr. Chasse found Constance drowsy but alert. When he asked why she had taken the overdose, she replied that she felt unusually depressed and believed that if taking a little medicine helped, taking a lot more would help her even further.

Chasse explained that such drugs did not work that way, and ordered Carl to flush the remainder of her medicines down the toilet. He then recommended that she see Dr. Stebbins, a psychiatrist in Bangor, as soon as possible.

Instead of seeing Dr. Stebbins, Carl opted to take her to a local psychiatrist, Dr. Paul Jones, who practiced in Union and the nearby Mansfield Clinic in Fairfield. On February 18, they had their first meeting with Dr. Jones at his clinic in Union.

After a brief visit, Jones assured Constance that those who talk about committing suicide seldom actually ever do. He told Carl and his mother Alice, who went to the appointment out of concern for the children, that there was no real cause for concern for his wife or the children. His final advice to Constance: "Go home and keep on with your work as a wife and mother."

In writing up the minutes of the appointment, Dr. Jones appeared confident in his diagnosis: **"Situational Depression brought on by their living condition at Snow Pond and the lack of a social life."**

He saw Mrs. Fisher again, this time on February 23, at the Mansfield Clinic in Waterville. It was a much more involved meeting. Constance was on a high or at her best. Or maybe she had already determined to kill herself and the children and it was all an act.

Jones wrote:

> *Her mood was decidedly light and she smiled and laughed frequently at appropriate times. She said she looked forward to the future and felt that now that they were living in town she would*

have more friends and that she would be able to get her husband to "go out more."

...she denied any periods of depression and thoughts of suicide saying "where do you suppose I got that idea? Probably I was just lonesome being at the camp and not seeing people."

But a new twist developed later that night when Jones returned to his practice in Union. He received a desperate phone call from Ursula Marcoux, saying that she had received in the mail something tantamount to a suicide note from Constance.

Jones wrote:

On arriving in Union that night I received a phone call from Mrs. Marcoux, the patient's foster mother.

She reported that she had received a note in the mail postmarked 11:30 a.m. (at which time the patient was in my office) The note gave direction as to where to find certain papers. The obvious implication was that the patient might destroy herself...

This report was so completely in variance with her appearance at the interview that I was at a loss to explain it to Mrs. Marcoux.

Carl Fisher was now running out of options. His wife's emotions would run the spectrum, and when she was down she was way down. At the advice of Dr. Fish at the Mansfield clinic, he considered sending her to the state mental hospital in Augusta.

But Constance objected and Carl was inclined to give in. She feared that if she was hospitalized there would be no one to properly care for the children. And even if she did become a patient at the Augusta State Hospital, could they really help her?

Carl had a problem. His wife would not comply with a voluntary commitment and she was not sick enough to be blue papered. He had little choice but to let a runaway train finish its course... or crash.

On top of her depression, Constance was once again being tormented by voices. At first she thought it might be God or of God, but now she wasn't sure. Would God want her to end the very lives she had brought into the world? And weren't both murder and suicide mortal sins, punishable by eternity in hell? And what about the commandment "Thou Shalt not Kill?"

Surely her priest, Fr. John F. Holihan would know. She planned to ask him but the appointment kept getting delayed.

On Ash Wednesday, the voice spoke to her again. And because this was a religious holiday, she concluded that it must be God after all. And the holiday was significant, Ash Wednesday. In the Bible, ashes were a sign of mourning, and only death causes mourning.

Having failed to do away with herself the first time, she heard the voice mocking her, calling her a coward, and threatening that things would only get worse. Day and night she conjured ideas of how to end her nightmare, ideas like inhaling exhaust fumes from the car, hanging herself, or stabbing herself with a knitting needle.

But now another idea roared full bloom into her head.

She needed to do away with her whole family, Carl included. Constance agreed with the voice that in the next life there would be an end to the awful nightmare that she perceived she and her family to be in.

Constance remembered a colt .45 automatic pistol that was kept at her parents' house. She had seen her foster father clean it a hundred times before putting it away in the top drawer of his bureau.

On the morning of February 17, knowing the Marcoux house would be empty, Constance trudged through the snow the short distance to 9 Riverview Road to steal the gun.

She let herself into the house, found the gun and clumsily forced a clip of bullets into the magazine, only to have the pistol misfire and discharge a bullet into the mattress. She fired again successfully into the mattress before sneaking out with the gun and returning to her apartment.

She would now wait for the right opportunity, at night while they slept, to murder her family. And then she would turn the gun on herself.

In the darkness, Constance Fisher roamed around the five- room apartment hour upon hour that night. The gun was loaded, and the safety was off, as she walked the floor wondering how she could ever follow through on such an awful plan. And for some reason, the voice was quiet, not urging or threatening as it had before.

By daybreak, Constance knew she could not go through with it. Somewhere deep in her conscience she knew that no matter how dark things might seem, she had no right to take the lives of her children and husband. She returned the gun the next day, only to steal it again two days later. But once again, she lacked the resolve to pull the trigger.

Monday, March 8, 1954 6:30 a.m.

Carl Fisher kissed his wife goodbye and grabbed the keys to his black Ford sedan for the short ride to the Maine Central Railroad terminus. From the bedroom window, Constance watched her husband put on his winter coat and hat and walk down the outside second story steps and enter the car.

For a moment, Constance lurched for the door to tell Carl that all was not well, that she was hiding a secret from him. That just days before she had brought a gun into the apartment to kill him and the kids. And that today she was going to kill herself and the children, just as the voice had commanded her.

But then she suddenly stopped, as if held by some unseen force.

For young Richard Fisher, it would be another day at school and he was having trouble adjusting. He had been attending the elementary school in Oakland, where he had lots of friends, and the school was within walking distance from his house on Snow Pond.

After Christmas break, however, his family had moved to Waterville and Richard was enrolled in the first grade at a new school, the Sacred Heart Catholic School in Waterville .

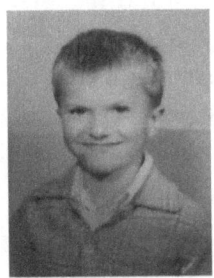

Richard "Dickie" Fisher
April 2, 1947- March 8, 1954
First Grade School photo
1953

It was a turbulent time for the youngster. It was a time of adjusting to a new teacher, new classmates and new neighbors.

School was a particular challenge. He had to make new friends in a strange place. The teachers, all females and nuns, looked imposing in their long black dresses and habits. Worst of all, he had to get used to wearing a school uniform, in which he felt awkward and funny.

But he had seen his dad in his military uniform. "Daddy" had served four years in the Air Force in World War 11 and was considered a hero for fighting despite contracting malaria and being wounded in battle, for which he received a medal. He was honored in the community, especially on Armistice Day, when he would wear his uniform and march in the parade.

Young Richard was the apple of his father's eye, his first born, the thought that gave him the sustenance to endure four years in an awful war. Slender and with green eyes like his father, Richard was named for his grandfather and would be the first Fisher to carry on the family name to a new generation.

To young Richard, the closest thing to God was his father, and the safest place on earth was at home with his mom and dad no matter where the physical location might be.

Then there was Richard's mom. To others it was Connie, Constance, Peggy, or Mrs. Fisher. But to Richard, she was "Mummy." There was never a question of her love and care. She rarely had a harsh word for any of the children and her affection was demonstrative, continually showering them with kisses and caresses.

And there was never accusation that any of the Fisher children where uncared for or denied anything materially or emotionally from their mother.

But young Richard must have known something was wrong with Mummy, as children instinctively do. There were her crying jags, days when she could scarcely get out of bed, and frequent trips to the doctor. She even had Daddy shoot the family pets. Yes, there was something wrong with Mummy; very wrong.

Although Richard excelled in his school work, being alone at recess while other groups of kids played was difficult. He tried hard to fit in with the other boys but it takes time. And time was not on his side.

At 3:00 on March 8, 1954 the final bell rang for the dismissal of school at the Sacred Heart Catholic School. Young Richard gathered his books, put his chair up on the desk and entered the line of students waiting for the school bus to take them home. Waiting at the door was Sister Dorothy who was bidding the children goodbye and a "see you in the morning."

The bus ride home was routine. It was a cold winter day and even the warmth of the school bus heater rattling full speed was nothing like it would be in just a few minutes at home. He sat alone. Even those who got off at the bus stop at the corner of High and Main Street were still strangers to him.

But soon he would be home where it would be warm, and Mummy would have a snack prepared for him as usual. And maybe Grammy or Aunt Louise or Uncle Billy would be there to play with him and Daniel and baby Debbie.

It seemed like they had been there a lot lately. And Daddy would be home at about 4:30. Maybe they could play with his baseball cards and talk about his favorite team, the Boston Red Sox, and his favorite player, Ted Williams. Williams, like Daddy, served in the Air Force. He too was a hero.

As the bus driver folded the doors closed, Richard stepped off the bus not knowing that the door to his life, open for such a brief span, would soon be shut by the most unlikely person in his world. The very person that had given him life was now waiting to take it.

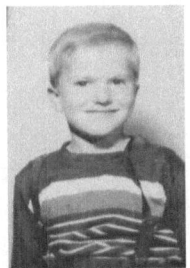

Daniel Brian Fisher
August 25, 1948- March 8, 1954
Kindergarten photo
1953

It was a short walk from the bus stop to the apartment. It was cold but the snow was turning to rain. The little sun light left was obscured by the clouds and the coming dusk. Hurriedly, Richard ran across the street and into the driveway of 31 High Street, skipping up the stairs to the family's second story flat.

Without effort he pushed the door open, and closed it behind him as he took off his coat and hat which he hung by the kitchen stove. As usual, Mummy was there to greet him. She held him in a long embrace.

Richard couldn't help but notice how quiet it was. He saw his brother Daniel lying on his bed wrapped in a blanket. His baby sister Deborah lay still in her crib.

"Son, get off your clothes and Mummy will draw you a warm bath."

He obediently entered into the bath tub, earlier the water grave of the two other Fisher children. As Constance began to bathe her child in the usual manner, she abruptly pulled him out of the water and gave him a long embrace before saying, "It will all be over soon, son."

Then she forced Richard under the water. Strong and wiry, he resisted his mother's efforts to drown him. "Mummy, what are you doing?" he yelled as Constance Fisher entered into the tub to complete the act. "It will be all right son, soon you will be in heaven."

Little Richard Fisher's last image was that of his first, of the woman who brought him into this world of joy and sorrow, pleasure and pain.

Φ Φ Φ Φ Φ Φ Φ Φ Φ Φ Φ Φ Φ Φ Φ Φ Φ Φ

HAVING NOW COMPLETED HER assignment, Constance Fisher wrapped the still bodies of her other two children in blankets and tucked them into their beds. But she had one task left to fulfill and the hour was getting late. Carl would be home shortly and she didn't want to be there when he arrived.

Hurriedly, she grabbed the bottle of Selsum Shampoo that Dr. Pratt had prescribed and drank from it till her innards burned. Then she wrapped herself in a blanket and slid under her bed to await the end.

But death would not come to relieve her suffering, a suffering that would only grow more acute in the days to follow.

At 4:00 p.m., the last trace of daylight was ebbing as Carl Fisher swung into the driveway. He noticed there were no lights on in the upstairs apartment. He hurried up the stairs and opened the door that was unlocked and entered the house.

There, he saw his second son, Daniel, lying motionless on his bed. He ran through the house hollering for his wife but got no response. He kicked open the locked bedroom door but she was not there.

He peered into the bathroom to find his son Richard, floating face down in the bathtub, apparently dead.

Frantic, Carl Fisher dialed Dr. Chasse who said he would be over immediately, and told him not to panic.

Accompanying Dr. Chasse was Constance Fisher's older sister Virginia, who was employed by Chasse as an assistant. Dr. Chasse insisted that she accompany him to the apartment.

"He made me come with him and kept telling me that whatever happens you're not going to break down," she later told police. "But after Dr. Chasse took the baby from her crib and put her in my arms, he just went to pieces."

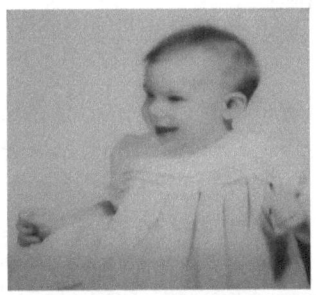

Deborah Kay Fisher
March 15, 1953-March 8, 1954
Age 9 months
1953

After touring the apartment, they found all the Fisher children, two in their beds, and the other, Richard, sprawled and face down in the bathtub. An unsuccessful attempt was made by Dr. Chasse to resuscitate him.

Absent, however, was Constance Fisher. Another search of the apartment found her under her bed, semi-conscious, and wrapped in an electric blanket. Beside her lay a bottle of Selsum Shampoo, its remaining contents puddled on the floor.

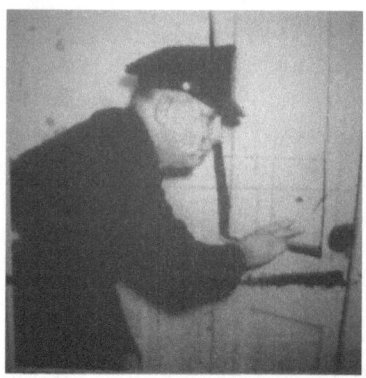

Patrolman Douris Beaulieu examines a door which the frantic father, Carl Fisher, battered when he found the two bodies of his children and sought desperately to find the third.
Waterville Sentinel, March 9, 1954. (2)

What exactly transpired on the morning of March 8, 1954 at the Fisher home was summed up in a report issued by the Waterville Police Department:

> *She drown the first child (Daniel) a little after 11a.m. She told Captain Drost that she told the child to take a bath. She played with him a while in the water, then hugged him and put him under the water. She had to get her head in the water in order to keep him down. When he was still she rolled him in a blanket and put him in his bed. Then she killed the baby by the same method.*
>
> *The six year old child came home about 3:30 p.m. With this one she had to hurry as she expected her husband home soon after 3:30. When she had him in the tub, she washed his feet and then started the same method. He looked up and said, "Mummy don't do that." She said, "it's all right, Richard, you'll be in heaven pretty soon." She got quite wet doing this.*
>
> *Then she had to hurry as she expected her husband home at any moment and she drank a small bottle, less than half a pint, of some kind of shampoo or hair tonic.*
>
> *She then took the electric blanket and pillows and got under*

the bed. She left the oldest in the bath tub, the baby in the crib in the master bedroom and the four year old in his room and she was under the bed of this child.

Her husband came home from work before 4 p.m. and, contrary to the newspaper record, did not find the door locked. He saw the four -year -old boy on his bed and couldn't tell immediately that he was dead. He shouted for his wife and had no answer. He ran to the shed door and found it locked. Then he ran to the bathroom and found the other boy. Then he rushed to Dr. Chasse and he came back with him and they found the mother under the bed.

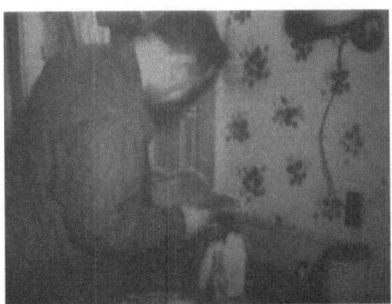

A note left by Constance Fisher at her High Street home in which she explained the reason for killing her three children, is read by Police Chief Albert Drost shortly after the bodies were discovered Monday afternoon. Waterville Sentinel, March 9, 1954.

Monday, March 8, 1954 5:00 p.m.

Constance Fisher covered her head with a towel and was escorted out of her home into the cold of the night by Captain Drost, Dr. Chasse, and her foster sister, Virginia Marcoux.

Other members of the Waterville police were called to the scene to take pictures and gather evidence. Patrolmen Douris Beaulieu and Russell Leblanc where the first to arrive, and seeing the scope of the tragedy summoned help from the Kennebec County Sheriff's office and the State Police.

The murder scene left an eerie tranquility. The family Bible lay open on the living room table. Children's slippers were drying near the kitchen stove. A play pen with dolls and a teddy bear lay motionless in the living room. Three quarts of milk were open and left on the kitchen table with cereal boxes and an unfinished cup of coffee.

On the kitchen table was a suicide note scrawled on the back side of a paper bag and addressed to Carl. It read, in part:

> *It was so hard to do it but God told me it was the only way I could save them. They are in heaven safe forever from evil... I hope you will forgive me- please forget all about us... maybe you don't think I loved them, I did, oh I did; my heart is breaking. I loved you and I loved them...*

The note also left detailed instructions about how Constance wished she and the children to be buried, and asked Carl to sell her rings to pay for the expenses. She urged her husband to go back and live with his mother.

Carl, who capsized under the horror of the incident, was given a sedative by Dr. Chasse and taken to the home of his parents who lived nearby in Oakland.

Mrs. Fisher was loaded into the police Cruiser that made its way through the snowy night to the Waterville Police station, where she was held for questioning.

By daybreak the city was abuzz with news about the tragedy. The Bangor Daily News for March 9, 1954 had a banner headline which read:

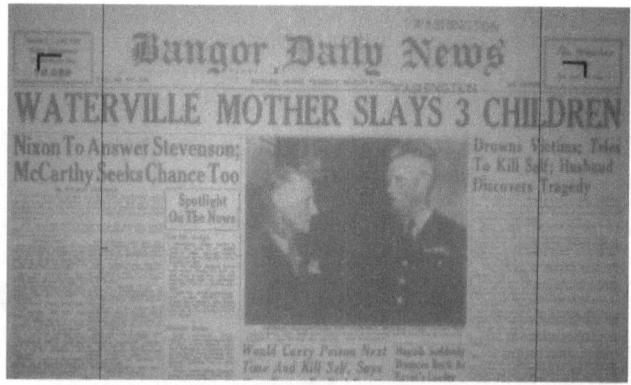

**Headline banner for the Bangor Daily News
Tuesday, March 9, 1954.**

Later in the week, the Waterville Sentinel gave this summation of its findings:

> *It was too late to avoid the tragedy she attempted to climax by taking her own life on Monday. Reliable sources said that Mrs. Fisher, fearing certain periodic nervous conditions herself had discussed the possibility of mental disorder with acquaintances and sought council of a psychiatrist. She was assured she had nothing to fear, according to reliable sources.*

And the story was rapidly spreading across the country. The Pittsburgh Post Gazette ran this brief:

> *A 24- year -old mother who left a suicide note saying her children are "in heaven safe forever from evil," was held today on suspicion of their murders.*
>
> *Kennebec County Attorney Joseph Campbell said Mrs. Carl Fisher had drowned Richard 6, Daniel 5, and Deborah 1, in the bathtub of their home yesterday.*
>
> *Mr. Campbell said that woman apparently attempted to take her own life by drinking a harmless scalp medicine but that it just left her dazed.*

Stunned, the Marcoux family circled the wagons and dedicated themselves to help Constance pick up the pieces in whatever way they could.

The family also rallied around the grieving father and husband. Carl Fisher would never return to the rented flat on 31 High Street. With the help of friends and relatives they loaded up the relatively few possessions and moved them to the home of his parents that would now become his residence for an indefinite period.

In her cell in the women's quarters of the Waterville city jail, Constance was visited by Kennebec County Attorney Joseph Campbell. The prosecutor told reporters that he was unable to learn all the details around the death or as to why two of the children were found in their beds.

"She blacks out on that," Campbell said. "All she can say is that God told me to do it."

Later that night she was interrogated again by Captain Drost, who found her weeping in the cell. She expressed that the only regret she had was that she had not succeeded in killing herself. Drost also learned that Mrs. Fisher had planned to murder her husband along with the children but couldn't find a gun.

Upon awakening in her cell on the morning of March 9, Constance Fisher began to realize the magnitude of her actions of the day before.

She was heard crying for about an hour by the police matron, Alice Simpson, who had no words that could console her. She refused breakfast, now knowing the events of the past 24 hours were not just a bad dream.

Shortly, she would face the legal system of the state of Maine that would determine her short and long- term fate. But first, she would have to face her husband who was escorted to her cell and given the opportunity to speak with her before the arraignment.

It can only be speculated what their conversation consisted of, although the jail matron reported loud cries, and sobs from Mrs. Fisher. She was next visited by her lawyer, Stanley F. Dubord who explained the legal options available to her.

She had the choice of a murder trial before a judge and jury who would render her innocent or guilty. Or, she could plead a defense that would allow her to acknowledge committing the crimes, but declare herself to be innocent by reason of insanity. At Dubord's insistence, she chose to plead not guilty by reason of insanity.

Her original court appearance was slated at noon but with an increasing amount of media and the curious buzzing around the court house, the hearing was moved to the afternoon.

At approximately 1:35 p.m., Constance Fisher was escorted through the underground tunnel that connected the holding facility to the municipal courthouse, to be arraigned on a murder charge.

Standing before Judge Arthur J. Cratty and a roomful of anxious on-lookers, Mrs. Fisher removed the handkerchief from around her face and wound it tightly around her hands. As she stepped before the bench, the clerk read the following charge against her:

> *… Constance Margaret Fisher did feloniously and willfully and of her malice and afterthought did kill and murder her three children.*

In a weak voice and with eyes closed she pleaded, "Not Guilty" to the charge.

Fifteen feet away sat her husband Carl. For most of the two- minute hearing he sat trembling, covering his face with his hands. When he heard his wife enter her plea, he put his hand over his mouth in an attempt to keep from sobbing.

Mrs. Fisher returned the handkerchief to her face, and covering her eyes, left the courtroom in the same manner she arrived.

She was then escorted to the Police Cruiser by Captain Drost, police Matron Alice Simpson and Deputy Sheriff Robert Donovan to be driven to the state hospital in Augusta for observation.

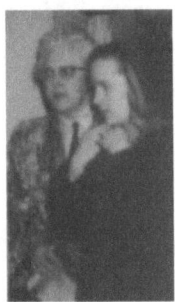

Mrs. Constance Fisher, charged with the bathtub murders of her three children, enters the Waterville County Courthouse prior to her arraignment Tuesday. Waterville Sentinel, March 10, 1954.

Mrs. Fisher left behind a city that was in shock about the nature and complexity of the crimes she had committed. In places of business, schools, and around family tables, residents were talking, wondering, and worrying about the event that shook the small, God-fearing community to its core.

Reaction oscillated from anger, to compassion, to sympathy, to outrage. Even a country hardened by the atrocities of a recent world war, had trouble digesting this loss of life.

Perhaps those most surprised were the people who knew Constance the best. Suicide? Maybe. Killing Carl and the kids? Unthinkable.

The psychiatric community was now being called upon to find some answers and they where gearing up for her arrival.

For sure, the doctors at the Augusta State Hospital were much more eager to see Mrs. Fisher than she was to see them.

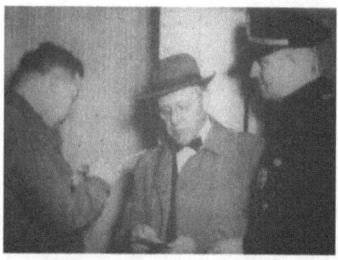

County and local authorities are shown at the scene of the triple murder of three young children shortly after the bodies were discovered. Waterville Sentinel, March 10, 1954.

* CHAPTER TWO *

BEGINNINGS

"Peggy was a stubborn child, but sensitive. She wouldn't hurt an ant."

Ursula Marcoux, 1954.

FROM THE VERY START, the life of Constance Margaret McConnell Sirois Fisher was shrouded in mystery.

As to who her biological parents were, Constance was never quite sure. But one thing was for sure; her biological parents never gave her any more than just a beginning.

A search of her birth record from the State of Maine Probate Court, provided the following:

> *The records of this court show the Adoption of Mary Teresa McConnell born in Norridgewock, Maine on March 26, 1929. The petitioners were Silvier F. Sirois and Rose T. Sirois of Bowdoinham, husband and wife. The child, Mary Teresa McConnell, according to the petition for Adoption, was the child of Madeline Sirois of Waterville, Maine and Albert McConnell and the petition recites that the "child is illegitimate, and the father of parts unknown." Consent to the adoption was given by Madeline Sirois, mother.*

... Spent the first year of her life as a Ward of the state, probably living in an institution or with a family member. The Decree of Adoption was granted on December 2, 1930, Silvier F. Sirois and Rose T. Sirois being the adopting parents, and the name of said child was changed to Mary Constance Sirois. (1)

Albert McConnell. Not much to be known about this obscure Mainer, although records hint that he spent most of his years moving from city to city in southern Maine.

The family's account was that McConnell had at sometime come to the city of Waterville or perhaps Bowdoinham, where he had a brief tryst with Madeline Sirois. The affair resulted in a pregnancy and the birth of Mary Teresa McConnell in 1929.

After the baby was born, McConnell was perhaps "encouraged" to leave by the Sirois family, or just shirked his responsibilities and drifted out of sight.

In 1930, according to the U.S. Census, McConnell was listed as living in Kittery at the homestead of George and Lydia Emmons. His occupation was stated as being in manufacturing.

McConnell then skipped from job to job, city to city, perhaps never knowing that his daughter would twice make national headlines. Or that his absence from her life may have been a major contributor to her problems. He died in Kittery at age 60 in 1967.

As for Madeline Sirois, relatives claim that she never left the Waterville area and never married. It is likely that she had no idea of what became of her baby.

The adoption practice in the state of Maine in 1929 was closed, and the birth parents and adoptive parents were not allowed to meet or share information.

All records and identities were sealed, including the baby's birth certificate. This effectively prevented the adoptive child and it's natural parents from ever finding each other.

It was thought that Madeline Sirois was a relative of Silvier Sirois, perhaps a niece, or a cousin from the extended family that had joined the great migration of French Canadians to Maine at the turn of the twentieth century.

At some point she moved to Waterville, and spent the rest of her life there, not far from the Sirois farm, and not far from the Marcoux property on Chase Street where Constance spent most of her childhood.

Being kin and living in proximity, they probably attended the same church, shopped at the same stores, attended the same family gatherings. One wonders how many times their lives intersected, all the while mother and child not knowing their intimate connection to each other.

Or maybe Madeline did know, and for that reason she stayed in the Waterville area. But what was the reason for her absence in Constance's life, especially at the times she was needed most? There is no record of her ever visiting Constance while she was a patient at the Augusta State Hospital.

Shortly after they were married, Carl stated that Constance raised the question of her parentage and wondered why her biological mother had never made an attempt to contact her. She concluded that her real mother had most likely committed suicide.

She and Carl made a singular attempt to travel to Norridgewock to find out exactly what had transpired but didn't find out much. Carl said that the subject was never broached again.

Mrs. Warren Marcoux, the only daughter of Silvier Sirois, who became the foster mother of Constance, had her own theory. Mrs. Marcoux stated that her father had but one brother, Eddie Sirois, who had a drinking problem that led his large family to move from place to place. She believed that Madeline was one of his children, one of the younger ones.

When the news arrived that young Madeline had given birth and the baby had become a ward of the state, Silvier was afraid someone from outside the family would get the child and agreed to adopt her.

Thus for the next two years, Mary Constance Sirois lived with her adoptive parents, Rose and Silvier who were now in their 60's. They split time between their farm in Bowdoinham and the Riverview Farm in Waterville.

The Riverview farm was a marvelous place to grow up with its barns filled with livestock and other animals more suitable for pets. There were big hay fields and ample fertile soil to raise acres of fruits and vegetables. The large parcel had its northern border on the Kennebec River, a wonderful place for outings and picnics, but ripe with dangers.

Over the years, its unforgiving, swift-moving currents had swept away the lives of many naive enough to enter its cold, dark waters.

But young Mary Constance would not spend long with the Sirois family. Rose died suddenly in the winter of 1932, leaving Silvier alone to raise the child. They stayed on the farm in Waterville the next year, until it was decided that they would live with the Marcoux family on Chase Street.

At that time, Warren and Ursula Marcoux were already trying to piece together a blended family of two children from Warren Marcoux's first marriage.

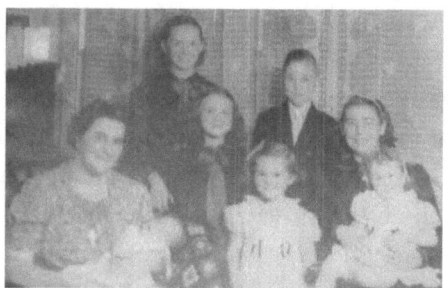

The Marcoux family c. 1940
Constance is standing, upper left.

At the age of 22, Warren Marcoux had unexpectedly found himself a widower. His wife died shortly after giving birth to a son, Robert, leaving a grieving parent alone to raise a son and a daughter. A dutiful family helped to fill in the gaps as best they could. But a young man needed a helpmate, and the handsome young businessman was sure to find someone.

But the respective fathers of Warren and Ursula, who knew each other through business, were not about to let nature takes its course. They arranged a meeting between the two, who quickly melded together like hand and glove. After a very brief courtship, they decided to get married.

They consulted the parish priest who dually noted the brevity of their relationship, but gave them his blessing saying "Go ahead. Those babies need a mother."

By 1935, both Silvier and Rose Sirois had passed away, leaving young Constance disenfranchised once again. Despite already rearing two children, with another on the way, Warren and Ursula Marcoux officially took Constance in as a foster child.

Warren and Ursula Marcoux went on to have seven more children. But death would be a frequent visitor at the Marcoux household.

They had a child that died still born. Three others died as infants due to Hydrocephalus, or water on the brain. Their five-year old daughter Natalie came in tired from play one day, and after falling asleep on her mother's lap, never awakened.

Although barely school age, Constance was deeply affected by the passing of her adoptive parents, to be followed by the death of three foster siblings. Added to the misery was the vexing question of, "Why would a loving God allow this?"

And where were the children now? Did they go to heaven to be with Rose and Silvier, both saints in her eyes? Or did they go to purgatory where the not-so-good, not-so-bad people end up? Or maybe they had done something really bad to cause their fate and were now suffering in Hell?

The parish priest quickly laid those fears to rest. The Catholic catechism said that because the children were not yet seven years old, they would go directly to heaven. And in Constance's mind, if that's what the Church taught then it had to be so.

Despite the turbulence of her first years, Constance fit in nicely with the rest of the Marcoux children. She was now the middle child, in between Virginia and Robert, and the three looked so much alike and were so close in age that they were often mistaken as triplets.

They had a camp on Messalonskee lake where they would spend wonderful summers swimming, fishing and exploring. And though these were the years of the Great Depression that would later transition into another World War, the Marcoux children never went without.

A strong Catholic faith was a pillar in the Marcoux household. Most of the kids were baptized and had their first communions and confirmations at the Sacred Heart Catholic Church in Waterville. Holidays and important dates on the church calendar were faithfully observed. The children attended parochial schools with the female children attending Mt. Merici, a private Catholic school for girls.

But for the Marcoux girls, there was not much thought about higher education. They were trained to be homemakers, learned cooking, sewing, and child-rearing. Their goals in life were those shared by most Catholic families of the day. They were expected to be good citizens, good parishioners, and good parents.

The Marcoux children had a strong father figure in Warren Marcoux, a hard-working, self made man who ran a prospering business. He was at first a car mechanic who later opened a GMC truck dealership in Waterville called Marcoux's Garage.

One of his first hires was his wife Ursula, who was the bookkeeper for the business. Intelligent, capable, and fluent in three languages, Ursula Marcoux could do anything she set her mind to. During the war years when family finances were down, she founded Kennebec Somerset Trucking Company. The business prospered and she later sold out to another company that became one of the largest truckers in New England.

But Ursula Marcoux was most happy fulfilling her call as a housewife and mother. And when the children fell short of her ambitions, "Mama" could wield the switch as well as anyone.

Often in need of the switch was young Constance. For most of her early childhood she had the unenviable position of being the middle child, the one that often slips through the cracks. And when the younger children came along, she fell even further down the pecking order.

Constance grew up in Waterville at a time when it was a heterogeneous manufacturing city of just under 10,000 persons. For such a small city, it was exceptional that her generation would produce, or host, several individuals that would earn national acclaim.

Among those were United States Senator George Mitchell, who brokered peace in Ireland and then was a special envoy to the Middle East. There was Dr. H. Richard Hornberger, a reputable surgeon, but much better known for his novel M*A*S*H and the spin off hit TV series of the same name.

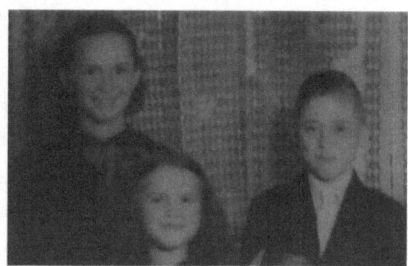

Triple threat. 1943
Constance was the leader of this gang of three.
Left to right, Constance, Virginia, and Robert.

The city was home to governors Clifford Claussen and Edmund Muskie. Muskie later became a United States Senator and U.S. Secretary of State, and was on track for a run for the Presidency in 1972.

It is probable that at one time or another, Constance rubbed shoulders with each of these, not knowing that each in their own way would leave a significant mark on history.

In her youth, Constance was described as care free, high-spirited, and always in hot water. Tomboyish, she fought with boys and girls alike, at least until she got her way. She could create sometimes hilarious mischief but was so soft-hearted that she didn't like anybody to hunt or fish, and was reluctant to crush even an ant.

The Marcoux children had a gang between them with Constance the unquestioned leader. She led them in and out of trouble, but mostly always in. She would often goad her siblings into testing the boundaries, like skating on a pond that was strictly forbidden or sneaking food out of the icebox.

Constance was also prone to pulling pranks, like putting the dishes in the washing machine, one time breaking a complete set of Mrs. Marcoux's favorite dishes and letting someone else take the fall for it. She could act impulsively, and fly off the handle at little things, but was said to never hold a grudge.

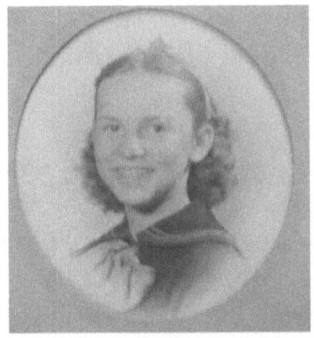

Constance Margaret Sirois in her early teens. High spirited and energetic, she made things interesting in the Marcoux household.

But Constance had another side, a more serious, introspective side. From an early age she pondered the great questions of life: Who am I? Why am I here? What purpose does my life serve? She kept a diary, journaled, and wrote poetry.

She could be quite introverted and rarely spoke about her problems. It seemed that little ruffled her feathers.

She could lose herself in a book, sometimes for hours as the rest of the children chummed and played. Like most teenagers, she was prone to day-dream, especially when there was house-work or school-work to be done.

Constance enjoyed all the intricacies of homemaking, especially needle work and cooking. She loved the outdoors where she could explore and enjoy all the marvels of nature and the companionship of pets and stray animals.

While she was said to be friendly to everyone, she had only a few close friends. She was faithful in her church attendance, and Christian development classes. She loved to dance and for a while wanted to study to become a ballet dancer.

When she became school age, Mrs. Marcoux enrolled Constance at Mt. Merici Academy, hoping that the nuns might add some discipline to the energetic, free-spirited child.

She entered Mount Merici Academy in 1934, and stayed there for four years. In 1938, she was transferred to Waterville Public Schools after Mrs. Marcoux tangled with school officials over the appropriateness of school uniforms.

She entered the fifth grade in the Waterville public school system, but was shortly demoted to the fourth grade for no apparent reason. Buford Grant, superintendent of schools added this addendum to her scholastic record:

> *In talking with the teacher she had, I find that she was not well adjusted and cried a great deal. On November 8th she was transferred to the fourth grade. No reason is given for this transfer. The records show no rank for the time she was with us therefore, I am unable to determine how she rated scholastically.*

With Mrs. Marcoux pregnant again, it was decided to send Constance away to a private Catholic boarding school. Maybe a mother's intuition was telling her that the child needed more attention than a very stretched Ursula Marcoux could give her.

Not quite ten years old, Constance boarded a train heading for the small Maine town of Jackman. She entered the Jackman Convent school at the mid-term on January 3, 1938.

Dorm-style living, and being away from home for the first time was yet another challenge for Constance. She was responsible to a matron nun who was assigned to instruct and nurture the child.

She lived on the second floor of a four-story brick building built at the turn of the twentieth century as a missionary outpost for the Catholic Church. The Convent complex consisted of the Sacred Heart Convent, that was home to clergy and boarding students, and the St. Anthony Parochial school.

There was not much to do in the logging community of about 1000 people, 16 miles from the Canadian border. There were no visitors allowed and relatives were only granted visits on holidays. But for Constance, it was the ideal situation to spread her wings and be free of sibling rivalries and house-hold chores. She was required to write and speak French and was academically challenged by the course work. And she became well-versed in the nuances of Catholic theology.

Her school-work at the Convent was considered satisfactory with her highest grades being in history, reading and religion. Special remarks on her report card ranged from "very commendable" and "showing improvement" to "appears not to try" and "capable of doing better".

Perhaps the most valuable lesson she learned at the convent was how to get along with the others in the tight confines of institutional living.

Having weaned her child, Mrs. Marcoux sent for Constance who returned home in the spring of 1941, and was re-enrolled at Mt. Merici.

Like the Jackman convent, Mt. Merici had originally housed a convent and later developed a K-12 school for parishioners. It was a highly respected institution in the community and known for its high academic and moral standards. The school emphasized it's own three R's; Respect, Responsibility, and Religion.

Because it was a private institution, it was considered a privilege to go to the school, and the students who did were often considered to be "uppity" or "holier than thou." Mrs. Marcoux was sure that none of her daughters got an attitude. She made them work twice as hard to appreciate the privilege.

Apparently, Constance performed well below her academic ability, and freely admitted that she did not try much in school. Her high school I.Q. test taken her junior year revealed a promising intellect and a mental age of 19.6. She sometimes thought of getting a college education, and maybe even becoming a doctor, but she knew that was out of the financial range of her parents.

In addition, they had already sent her to a private boarding school. For a while she felt that she might want to be a psychiatrist…

High school brought with it the emotional and physical changes that most adolescents fight through. The physical changes transformed the tomboy into an attractive young woman. When quivering male voices began to ask for her on the telephone, she was often chided and teased by her siblings.

It was said that Constance was the most attractive of all the good-looking Marcoux girls, and that she had charm and a quick wit. By her Junior year she began to excel in her academics and had more than her fair share of admirers and suitors.

During high school years, Constance often chummed with her foster brother, Robert, who landed her a job as a baker's helper at the Harris Baking Company in Waterville. They both worked the morning shift from 4:00 am to 8:00 am before heading to school.

Unfortunately, Constance's high school career would be cut short before her graduation date, set for June of 1946.

A chance meeting with a returning air force sergeant changed her senior year and her life in the fall of 1945.

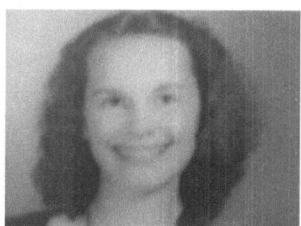

Constance at 17.
This would have been her graduation picture from
Mount Merici had she stayed in school.

Carl Merrill Fisher had recently returned to the nearby town of Oakland after receiving an honorable discharge for his service in the Air Force.

Like many of the returning Vets, Carl was eager to find a wife, build a home, and start living the American dream that he had risked his life to protect.

It was uncertain where they met, maybe at the Harris Bakery Company where Constance sometimes worked the counter, or maybe at the Dance Pavilion in Oakland, a popular hang-out for young adults and high school students.

It must have been true that opposites attract. There were stark differences between Constance and Carl. Most obvious was the age difference of nine years. Carl at 25 had the maturity of a war veteran who had seen the world and tasted of combat.

Constance had the naivety of star-struck teenager. She was still a student in a cloistered Catholic high school, and had scarcely ventured beyond the borders of her own backyard.

Carl was subdued, calculating, serious. Constance, energetic, life of the party, and spontaneous. From the start, if Carl was the drink, Constance was the straw that stirred the drink.

Around Christmas of 1945, after knowing each other a few scant weeks, Carl proposed, and without as much as an arm's twist Constance accepted. A wedding date was set for June of 1946, right after her graduation from Mt. Merici.

But the situation ran into a snag. Because Constance was now engaged, the principal at Mt. Merici would not allow her to return for the last half of her senior year. Although Constance could have finished her education at nearby Lawrence High School, she opted instead to go to work full time for the Harris Baking Company and save up some money for her wedding.

A letter sent as part of her transcript summed up Constance's time at Mount Merici:

> Enclosed is a duplicate of Constance Fisher's high school record. You will notice that her grades are much below her mental ability.
>
> Mrs. Fisher was a passionate reader and spent every free moment of her high school days reading. For that reason, she was not considered very sociable and was not a good mixer.
>
> According to our records, Constance registered with us in September of 1934 and remained until January of 1938. She

came back in September of 1938 and remained until June of 1945. She maintained a B average through the grades. Her health was good. She was a little difficult to handle because of her stubborn nature.

Your truly,
Mother St. Arsene, O.S.U
Principal

The suddenness of their marriage was not uncommon at the time. The returning veterans were considered a good catch with their paid college education, interest-free housing loans, and honored place in the community.

At first Warren and Ursula Marcoux had some misgivings about the brief courtship and impending marriage.

Only 17, they figured that Constance was hardly ready to take on the responsibilities of pleasing a husband, tending a household and raising a family. And what about the untapped potential of the underachieving student whose I.Q. testing had bordered on genius?

But the Marcoux's were impressed with Carl, feeling his mature, calming influence would be of great benefit to their daughter.

Although counseled by her parents to wait, Constance succumbed to her impetuous nature. It was a mistake of course. She would later admit, "I was married way too young; I needed a father more than a husband."

Carl Merrill Fisher and Mary Constance Sirois were married on Saturday morning, June 26, 1946, following a wedding breakfast held at the Marcoux residence.

The ceremony was simple and of course Catholic. It was held at the Sacred Heart Catholic Church in Waterville, where the Marcoux family attended and Carl had recently become a member.

The service was held in the company of a small crowd of family and friends. Providing music was Virginia Marcoux, who ironically sang the Ava Maria, Mary's consolation ode at the loss of her child, Jesus.

Constance wore a pale gray suit with pink accessories carrying a gray prayer book intertwined with roses and buds. She stood beside Carl and his father, Norman Fisher, as Rev. John F. Holohan read the couple the most binding element of their wedding vow:

"To be faithful in sickness and in health, For better or for worse..."

As none can, the couple hadn't an inkling of what those words would one day entail.

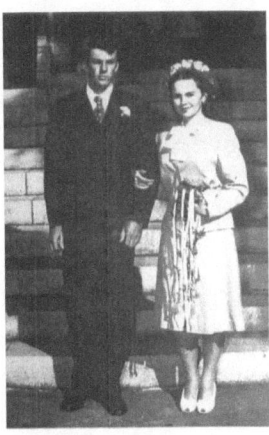

Wedding day, Saturday, June 26, 1946
"If ever a man was tested by his wedding vows it was Carl Fisher."
Dr. Ulrich Jacobsohn

Just before noon, the newly-weds took off in Carl's 1946 black Ford sedan for the Fishers' hunting lodge in Beddington, to be followed by a honeymoon trip to Augusta to view the state capitol.

Carl and Constance began their new life together in Oakland where Norman Fisher had set up an efficiency apartment for them.

The couple had one big advantage starting off. Because of the benefit of the GI Bill, Carl could attend for free the University of Maine in nearby Orono, or any number of technical schools.

He had one problem, however. He hadn't finished high school either.

It really didn't mater anyway. Carl was good with his hands and knew he could make a way for himself. He soon found work as a carpenter and then as a box car builder at the Central Maine Railroad yard.

Initially, Constance was elated with the freedom from the restraints of her foster parents. She and Carl enjoyed each other's company and would often enjoy the nightlife in nearby Waterville, and sometimes travel into Augusta as they did on their honeymoon.

Constance's freedom was short-lived, however. Although the couple had wanted to wait and become financially stable before starting a family, she conceived shortly after her wedding night and on April 2, 1947 gave birth to a son.

The extended family had eagerly awaited the birth of Richard, a handsome blonde-haired, green-eyed child, beloved by both sets of grandparents and scattered aunts and uncles. Richard was followed by Daniel, and then a daughter, Deborah.

Both sides of the family were wonderful to the young couple. And they adored the children, showering them with gifts at Christmas, birthdays and any other excuse. The Fisher and Marcoux families blended nicely, spending vacations and holidays together and often gathering after church on Sunday.

And there was always money available from in-laws in a pinch. With Constance a full-time mother and Carl not earning much more than $50 a week, things could get tight on occasion.

In 1950, Carl bought a cabin on near by Snow Pond, spending long hours after work to make it livable for his family. Although primitive in some respects, it had all the essentials, and the asture lifestyle appealed to the adventuresome aspect of Constance's personality. They both treasured the privacy that it offered, although the days often became lonely for Constance with no one to talk to but the kids and the pets.

Constance seemed to blossom as a young housewife. She was industrious and loved to work around the camp making it into a home. She was clever with her hands, liked to knit and make the children's clothes and her own gifts for people. In charge of the family budget, she learned how to make the most out of Carl's meager paycheck.

But she dreamed about the day when she and Carl could afford a real house, a farm out in the country with animals, gardens, and a pond. Just like it was when she was a child living with Rose and Silvier.

Every Sunday after church there was a big gathering of the extended family at the Marcoux house, with the Fisher children being the center of attention. The soft-spoken Carl would exclaim while the children bounced on his lap that the best thing in the whole wide world was family, and that he had the best.

And Carl and Constance seemed like they had the ideal family with three beautiful children, and a life somewhere between Ricky and Lucy, and Ozzie and Harriet.

And with a loving extended family to support them, the future looked bright, until something went wrong… terribly wrong.

CHAPTER THREE

A NEW HOME

"We visited the Lunatic Asylum on the east side of the river in this town... and were surprised to find so capacious and noble a building. It is an honor to the humane spirit of our state."

The News Teller, June 23, 1840.

IT WAS A WARM day in central Maine on March 11, 1954, displaying a glimmer of early spring.

Dirty melting snow banks lined the roads while small glaciers melted in parking lots. Long barren trees were beginning to show buds. Lawns were a patch-work of brown and white spots with a whisper of green that hinted of the comming spring.

Most Mainers waded through the day still dressed in winter garb, hoping spring would come sooner than later. But for Constance Fisher, spring or not, the outlook was as dark as a cold winter night.

It is hard to imagine what was going on in her mind during the 35-mile drive from the Waterville Municipal Court building to the Augusta State Hospital, her new home for the foreseeable future.

She was now perfectly lucid. She was aware of the fate of her children, and the extent of the grief she had caused her loved ones. And the anxiety about the world she would enter in a very few minutes was beginning to show.

At 3:45 p.m. the cruiser pulled onto Arsenal Street, and a complex of stone and brick buildings began to appear which comprised the state's chief mental health institution. Mrs. Fisher was escorted by Captain Drost and two matrons into the Stone Building, an imposing granite structure, where she would be admitted, given a bed, and await evaluation.

For all she knew, she might never leave the complex once she entered. Or maybe she would end up in prison, or maybe she would be executed. Her prospects were as uncertain as the changing Maine weather.

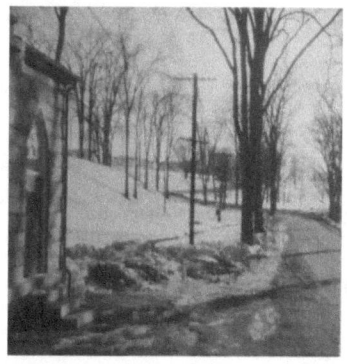

1950's view from the gatehouse at the Augusta State Hospital. It would be the same view that Constance Fisher had from the back seat of the police cruiser on March 11, 1954 looking up Arsenal street as she entered the Augusta State Hospital. Courtesy Maine Historic Preservation

There would be no electric chair for Mrs. Fisher or lethal injection. The death penalty had been outlawed in Maine in 1877 following the grizzly death of escaped convict Daniel Wilkinson, who was put to death by hanging.

If found guilty of the murder of her three children, Constance Fisher could be sentenced to life in prison and sent to the women's correctional facility in Skowhegan. Or if found innocent by reason of insanity, she could be committed to the Augusta State Hospital for the remainder of her life.

But a recently amended law stated that in the event that Mrs. Fisher could be helped at the hospital to the point that she was no longer a threat to herself or the community, she could be released. (1)

But first she would be evaluated, not treated, to see if she was fit to stand trial for the murders of which she was the only suspect.

As the cruiser pulled up to its destination, Mrs. Fisher's thoughts turned to Carl.

She knew he must be entirely devastated. Not only had he just lost his children, but for all practical purposes his wife. In the space of 24 hours, his plans and dreams for the future had melted as fast as a snowball on a hot summer day.

Perhaps it would have been better for Carl if she had succeeded in her attempt at suicide; at least he would have closure and a chance to start anew. But now he shared her uncertain fate at the hands of the medical and judicial authorities.

But Carl's thoughts were elsewhere. Tomorrow he would lead a solemn procession that would make its way to the southern end of the St. Francis's Catholic Cemetery in Waterville. There his three children whom he loved more than life itself would be interred along with a piece of his heart.

He was joined at the site by his parents, Norman and Alice, brothers David, Paul, Robert, and sister Helen. The Marcoux family and close relatives also came to grieve and show their support.

Carl's grief was extraordinary. Even all his military training and experience were inadequate for the moment. His progeny had been cut down, not by enemy fire, but by the one he loved and trusted most.

The three white caskets glistened in the sun for a moment before they were lowered into the ground. Hidden beneath the earth, yes, but never to be forgotten by this grief-stricken father.

Perhaps for a moment Carl Fisher wished that Constance had succeeded in her initial plan of killing them all.

Φ Φ Φ Φ Φ Φ Φ Φ Φ Φ Φ Φ Φ Φ Φ Φ Φ Φ

STANDING UNDER THE LARGE porch between the gothic columns that lined the entrance to the Stone Building, Constance Fisher was now led up the granite steps and into the admissions area where she was admitted and given a brief physical examination.

Despite the admonition by the hospital's top administrator, Dr. Francis Sleeper, that Mrs. Fisher be treated as any other patient, there was a buzz of excitement and alarm throughout the hospital with the news of her arrival.

As in any social setting, there was a certain aristocracy at the hospital, especially among the patients. And those who were at the hospital for abusing their children were on the lowest rung of the ladder. But Constance Fisher had taken that a giant step further. She had killed hers.

For the first 30 days, Constance was assigned a bed in the observation area that was kept locked with 24- hour suicide watch. Considered to be harmless to everyone but herself, she was then assigned to a ward in Middle Stone, the oldest portion of the original building in the complex.

The imposing four-story granite building had wards for both male and female patients. It's simple, resilient architecture was built for the long haul, expressing the determination its inhabitants must possess if they were ever to leave.

The Stone Building was the centerpiece of an array of buildings, close to seventy in all, that comprised the hospital. In many ways the Augusta State Hospital resembled a college campus with it's differing components melded together over years of growth to form a single entity and a common purpose.

And there were other parallels between the hospital and a college campus:

> *Occupants were part of a heterogeneous population.*
> *Occupants lived in an institutional setting.*
> *Occupants needed to master the art of being an individual in a community setting.*
> *Occupants needed to give up certain rights and freedoms in order to attain their goals.*
> *Occupants developed a camaraderie with fellow humans at a similar station in life.*
> *Occupants would sometimes exhibit deviant and /or irrational behaviors.*
> *Occupants used drugs.*

Occupants were given no guarantee for success.

Occupants had a significant suicide rate.

Occupants learned that it was the patient or the student who determined their ultimate success, not the physician or the professor.

And while the college student worked to earn a degree to secure employment in the outside world, the hospital patient worked to re-gain health and find a place back in society.

Unfortunately, for some patients graduation could take decades. Others might never graduate, spending the rest of their lives at the institution.

But for those who would never improve enough to leave, at least they had a place to call home where their basic needs were met. There, they could feel a sense of safety and security they would not enjoy if forced back on the outside. They had good food, free medical care, and recreational activities. Indeed, the majority of Maslow's hierarchy of needs were, or could be, satisfied at the hospital. (1)

For the many who would stay, it was a drastic improvement over the situations they had left. At the hospital they had a refuge from the dysfunctions that often exaggerated their illness rather than relieve it.

The argument was made however, that despite the care and opportunities offered, the patients were not "free" while committed to the institution. Free? What is free?

The great irony is that patients treated at the Augusta State Hospital in the 1950's had a greater freedom and quality of life than many of those who lived in other gated communities, like Palm Springs.

Those on the outside, including the rich and famous, have their own dysfunctions, often self-medicating with drugs, alcohol, and other chains. They are not "free" either.

Φ Φ Φ Φ Φ Φ Φ Φ Φ Φ Φ Φ Φ Φ Φ Φ Φ Φ Φ

SINCE ITS BEGINNING, THE Augusta State Hospital had an emphasis on treating the patient, not on punishment, confinement or simply warehousing people. It was to be a place where the de- humanizing chains of mental illness could be broken or perhaps loosened. It was a hospital first and foremost, and the expectation was that patients would get well and return to their families and communities as quickly as possible.

Its message was to proclaim that mental illness is just that, not a character flaw or a moral failure. And like any other illness, it could be treated and cured.

The hospital was free to any citizen in the state in need of its services, but because the State of Maine was its primary benefactor, the hospital would be at the mercy of the legislature to appropriate adequate funding for its operation.

Historians say that the site selected for the hospital was intentionally aligned so that every time the legislature and the governor looked out their eastern view windows, they would have a direct view of the hospital.

It was the same device used in building most of the countries earliest colleges. Divinity schools at first, the campus was laid out with the chapel as the focal point, so that at every turn there would be a reminder that God was the center, inspiration, and foundation of all knowledge.

It was the legislators, who in proxy for the citizens, determined if there would be enough beds to accommodate the patient population. Their votes determined the quality of care, and if there would be sufficient staffing to carry out the goals and objectives of the physicians.

They became the de facto social conscience of the state. It was they who determined the extent of the care provided for "the least of these."

Unfortunately, they did not always make wise choices.

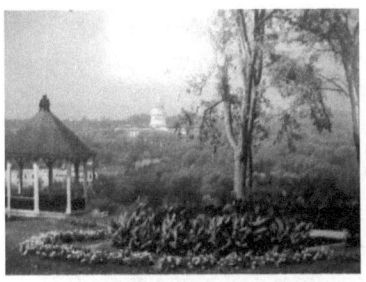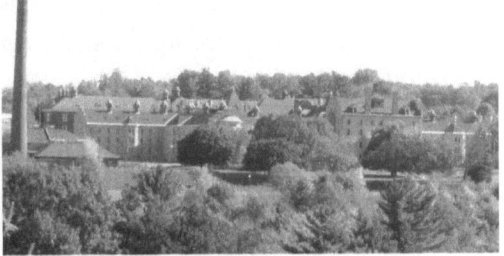

Two views of the Augusta State Hospital
Left: A post card view of the state capital as seen from
the grounds in front of the Stone Building.
Right: The view of the hospital as seen from the eastern
window of the Maine House of Representatives.

Alice Frost Lord, a reporter for the Lewiston Journal Magazine, wrote of the contrasting views in 1937.

> *"Strange to stand in the beautiful granite porch of the Augusta State Hospital and look across the Kennebec River to the western shore and see rising skyward one of the noblest capitol domes in the country.*
>
> *What contrast between the purposes of these two State institutions that so confront each other…two extremes dropped into the valley, with but a river between them. How narrow that which separates the two. And how beyond the power of any individual to predetermine his birth right, or to a great extent the circumstances which may lead him to the one side or the other!"*

The erection of the Maine Insane Hospital was quite a sensation to Mainers living in the late 1830's. After the state capitol building, it was the second building built by the state, and one of the original 13 hospitals for the mentally ill in the nation.

An area newspaper, The Augusta Age, had this to say about the new hospital:

> *If any citizen or stranger in this town has a leisure hour let him visit the building now erecting for the purpose of an insane hospital. We doubt whether many, even of our own citizens are aware of the magnitude of the work or the unsurpassed beauty of the location… Of the admirable arrangement of the*

building, and its complete adaptation to the noble purpose for which it is intended we have not time or space to speak half of this observation.

Hayward's New England Gazetteer wrote:

The State Insane Hospital. This splendid granite edifice is an honor to the state and to humanity. It occupies a plot of elevated ground of seventy acres on the east side of the river. Its situation is unrivalled for the beauty of its scenery. This building was commenced in 1836 and will probably be completed and prepared to receive patients in 1839. It will cost the state and some beneficent individuals who have made liberal donation towards its erecting about $100,000. It is of the model of the lunatic hospital at Worcester, Mass.

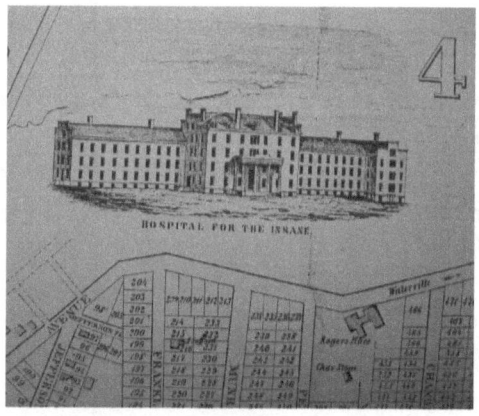

**Architects rendition of the new insane hospital in Augusta
c. 1835
Courtesy Maine Historic Preservation.**

While planners looked toward Massachusetts for its design, they looked towards Vermont for its treatment mode.

In Brattleborough was a hospital that was gaining national and international acclaim as a model in the treatment of the mentally ill.

Founded in 1834, the physicians at the institution insisted that mental illness was neither predestined nor incurable, and that if given the right environment and treatment, mental illness could be contained and cured as well as any physical illness.

It used a working farm, newspaper, gymnasium, camping program, swimming pool, bowling alley, golf course and even a 70-meter ski jump to give patients a reprieve from their illnesses while attempting to re-train their thought processes.

As early as 1830, Maine had been moving in a similar direction, considering it a crime against humanity to ignore the plight of the men-tally ill. That year, Governor Jonathan Hunton asked the legislature that provisions be made for a building exclusively for the treatment of the mentally ill.

In August of 1830, a questionnaire was sent out to the postmaster of every town in Maine, asking "How many insane and how many id-iots do you have in your town?"

Based on the data received, it was determined that statewide 562 in-dividual were deemed insane or about one in every three hundred res-idents. The report said that many of the ill had been banished to back rooms and barns. Others lived as unwanted vagabonds being driven from town to town. Many were incarcerated in jails, prisons, and poor houses.

Reports and statistics however, failed to adequately tell the story of the mentally ill in Maine before there was a hospital able to care for them.

The Maine Insane Hospital report of 1840 gives a ghastly snapshot of the institution's clientele and the awful conditions from which they were retrieved:

> *Among the incurable cases admitted during the year, a large proportion were of the most disagreeable kin, noisy, violent and filthy from years of confinements in cages and similar contrivance, that had divested them of every pleasing attribute of nature.*
>
> *... some of them the severity and duration of their disease aided perhaps by unskillful and heartless management, have con-verted into the most wretched and repulsive objects that bear the human form.*
>
> *Their occasional violence inspiring fear, they were perpetually confined in cages or dungeons, where their feelings are lacerated by unkindness and their most animal wants are uncared for. In*

> *those wretched abodes no light of heaven streams upon their eyes,*
> *the genial warmth of fire is never felt and seldom does the cheering*
> *voice of a fellow man sound upon their ears.*
>
> *For want of other occupations to engage their attention and*
> *consume their nervous energy, they drag out their existence wal-*
> *lowing in filth or rending the air with their vociferations. This is*
> *no fancy picture, but the plain uncolored reality. (2)*

The scope of the atrocity of this un-addressed problem stood over-whelming to most Mainers. But with a renewed interest in being "your brother's keeper" fueled by the second Great Awakening, and the recognition that mental illness might be curable, Mainers became an example to the rest of the nation by building a state of the art hospital exclusively for the mentally ill.

Cyrus Knapp, the first superintendent of the Maine Insane Hospital, had this to say of the new enterprise:

> *The building was ready for the reception of patients on the*
> *14th of October last. For neatness of workmanship, strength, dura-*
> *bility and the adeptness to the purpose for which it was designed,*
> *it may advantageously compare with any public building in the*
> *country.*
>
> *In its plan and finish, nothing that could contribute to the*
> *connivance of the officers, or to the comfort, safety and restora-*
> *tion to health of the patients, seems to have been forgotten or*
> *neglected...*
>
> *Convinces for bathing, showering and preserving in every*
> *way among the patients personal cleanliness, are furnished in ev-*
> *ery gallery. The building on the whole, is an honor to the state.*

Dr. Knapp went on to explain that those entering the hospital were patients, not inmates, itself a revolutionary concept. Knapp spoke of establishing a therapeutic community in which the habits learned by the suffering individual, often the result of a dysfunctional or abusive environment, could be corrected if given a literal change of scenery.

He stressed that patients must be intellectually stimulated and kept busy with physical labors. Working in the fresh air and sunshine, male patients would do farming or tend animals, and be rewarded by a restful night sleep and a feeling of accomplishment. Female patients would spend their time in such familiar tasks as sewing, knitting and laundering.

Knapp also began acquiring a small library with books carefully screened to promote wholesome thought. The library was greatly enhanced by the gift of Dr. Benjamin Vaughan, who donated his medical library to the institution, which was thought to be the best collection in New England, if not the country.

Besides physical exercise in the fresh air and sunshine, cleanliness was also required. Knapp wrote:

> *The abundant supply of water and means of ventilation afford ample faculties for carrying into effect the most rigid rules of cleanliness and purity of air, which we regard as indispensable requisites in the successful management of the institution. Much attention is devoted to the personal cleanliness of the patient and the neatness and comfort of their clothing.*

In acquiring the "abundant supply of water" through the wells and cisterns dug on the property, Knapp had unknowingly tapped the aquifer that was feeding the springs at nearby Togus, now becoming nationally renowned for their curative powers.

Knapp noted the patients had emotional and spiritual needs that need to be recognized and addressed. He wrote:

> *In all our intercourse with the patients we treat them with the most careful attention, gentleness and kindness and they readily learn that we are their friends and protectors.*
>
> *Thus treated, the raving and violent become calm and their gloomy and despondent mood turns cheerful giving an opportunity for the light of reason to be rekindled in the mind and the general health to be restored.*
>
> *Nearly all of our patients attend the daily evening religious services conducted in the Hospital and almost with out exception manifest much pleasing in the subject.*

The concept of Sabbath or rest, was also employed. Newly admitted patients were encouraged to rest, mentally and physically, that their excited systems might relax and have a chance to regain equilibrium.

And sleep, the great restorer, was also acknowledged as the great equalizer. During sleep hours, which constitutes almost 1/3 of a life span, there is no difference between the king on his throne and the prisoner in his dungeon.

Under Knapp, and then Dr. Isaac Ray, the institution began to codify rules of admittance and behavior. The following are examples taken from the superintendents report of the period:

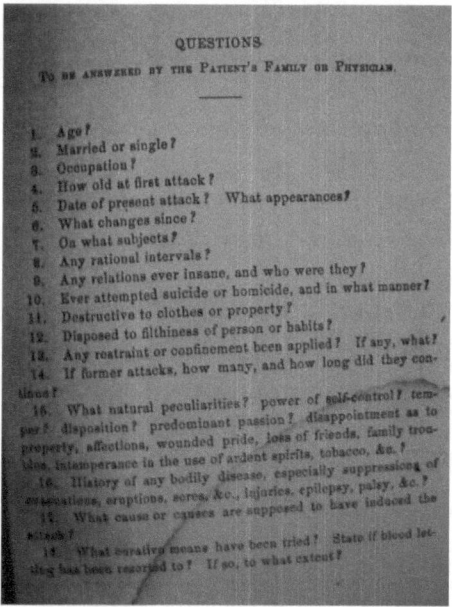

QUESTIONS

To be answered by the Patient's Family or Physician.

1. Age?
2. Married or single?
3. Occupation?
4. How old at first attack?
5. Date of present attack? What appearances?
6. What changes since?
7. On what subjects?
8. Any rational intervals?
9. Any relations ever insane, and who were they?
10. Ever attempted suicide or homicide, and in what manner?
11. Destructive to clothes or property?
12. Disposed to filthiness of person or habits?
13. Any restraint or confinement been applied? If any, what?
14. If former attacks, how many, and how long did they continue?
15. What natural peculiarities? power of self-control? temper? disposition? predominant passion? disappointment as to property, affections, wounded pride, loss of friends, family troubles, intemperance in the use of ardent spirits, tobacco, &c.?
16. History of any bodily disease, especially suppressions of evacuations, eruptions, sores, &c., injuries, epilepsy, palsy, &c.?
17. What cause or causes are supposed to have induced the attack?
18. What curative means have been tried? State if blood letting has been resorted to? If so, to what extent?

> ## GENERAL DIRECTIONS.
>
> Every patient must be in charge of some responsible individual at all times, unless permitted to be at large by the Superintendent. And when taken from the galleries by any person, that person is responsible for their safe keeping till returned to the halls, or entrusted by the officers to the care of another.
>
> No patient is permitted to go out of the wings without the consent of the officers, and no new patient without the order of the Superintendent.
>
> The whole time of all the attendants and assistants belongs to the Institution. This does not prohibit each individual from attending to his or her clothing; but to no other service can they devote any time ; nor can they receive any compensation for their labor, excepting their regular wages, but by express permission of the Superintendent in each case.

Clinicians at the Maine Insane Hospital in the 1840's were by no means fighting a new enemy. It is apparent that mental illness has vexed the human race since the beginning, but at least now they were fighting it, not ignoring or punishing it.

One of the earliest manuscripts of recorded human history, the Bible, contains evidence that mental illness plagued the cradle of civilization.

The Scripture records that Israel's King David feigned madness to escape the hand of Achish, King of Gath.

When David was presented to Achish, the king replied, "Behold you see this man behaving as a madman. Why do you bring him to me? Do I lack madmen, that you have brought this one to act like one in my presence? Shall this one come into my house?" (3)

Achish's response was significant, and sadly prophetic: Get these people out of my sight, and away from me.

Some of the earliest beliefs about mental illness were that evil spirits possessed victims and relief was sought by drilling a hole in the victim's head to let the spirits escape. Others in the ancient world endured treatments such as murder, dismemberment and confinement.

Over time, some strides were made only to be lost and re- found again by another generation.

Hypocrites believed that mental illness was the result of a chemical imbalance in the body and therefore could be treated. He cited depression as an example of an excess of black bile or "melan chole," the origin for the English word melancholy.

The Greeks and the Romans treated mental illness as they did bodily illness with blood-letting and a host of homeopathic remedies. And they were much more civil to the mentally ill than others of antiquity, even granting a criminal defense based on insanity or mental impairment.

The treatment of the mentally ill lapsed back into superstition during the middle ages, when people exhibiting symptoms of mental illness were considered to be witches and were burned at the stake, hanged, or drowned. The same held true in colonial America, giving way to the Salem Witch Trials.

Sentiment among the common folk of the colonial period was driven by the unfounded notion that once mentally ill or insane, always insane. Or that they were under judgment for their sins and should be left alone to bear their sufferings.

Neither was there a distinction between criminal behavior and mental illness. In 1683, a depressed Dorothy Talbye was hanged for murdering her daughter, the first recorded case of filicide in the new world.

The insane were divided into two categories, the dangerous and the harmless. Strong houses were built in the town squares to accommodate the most severe cases where they were regularly taunted. "Baiting the Looney" became a popular pastime in many American communities.

Others found their way into the town jails where they lived with criminals and murderers with no provision for the separation of sexes.

Those not incarcerated banded together like lepers seeking refuge by moving from town to town. In some towns they would be auctioned off to the highest bidders, bought like chattel in town meetings or the local tavern.

Later, statute mandated that responsibility must be taken by towns for those incapable of caring for themselves. This only succeeded in putting more ailing people in jails or prisons where the care was cruel and futile. Others were loaded in the dead of night in carts and dumped off in other towns.

But early in the 19th century, the notion came that the mentally ill were conscious of their emotions, capable of feeling, and perhaps even curable. The reform movement of the early 19th century finally took the plight of the mentally ill out of the dark ages.

The new focus was on curing instead of containing. Groups like the Quakers were among the first to espouse this concept and in 1813, opened a hospital in a setting that removed the shackles and opened the doors to humane treatment.

In 1810, Dr. Benjamin Rush, the father of American Psychiatry, established what was to become a model for new hospitals springing up in the U.S. and abroad. His book, "Inquiries of the Diseases of the Mind" was the first psychiatric textbook printed in America. He lectured his students who would become doctors to "attend to the poor, they are your best patient. God is their pay master."

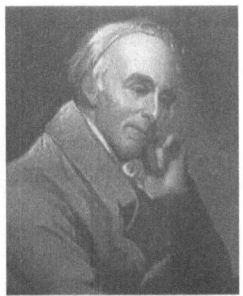

Dr. Benjamin Rush.
Reformer, Scientist, and Author.

In his hospital in Pennsylvania, Rush took a holistic approach to the treatment of mental illness. He began to move the setting to the fresh air and pleasant surroundings of the suburbs, where work, amusements, and exercise became an important part of the treatment. Essential to his plan was getting patients out of the very environment that had caused and was increasing their illness.

Individual wards separated the harmful patients from less harmful ones, males from females, and differentiated degrees of illness. He found funding to hire capable and qualified staff. Occupational and recreational treatments were provided and patients were kept clean, neat and given an adequate diet. He insisted that the building have lots of natural light, fresh air and pure drinking water.

The concept of the building and grounds as being part of the treatment was furthered by another Philadelphia doctor, Thomas Kirkbride.

Kirkbride believed the building should promote privacy and comfort for patients and that the grounds should be attractive and engaging.

The Kirkbride plan called for a picturesque location that provided an ideal environment to promote healing and tranquility to its often tormented tenants.

The treatment plan advocated by Rush and later Dr. T. Romeyn Beck became known as "Moral Treatment" and institutions employing this treatment mode had unprecedented success across the U.S. and Europe.

The moralists believed that mental illness grew out of a violation of physical, mental, and moral law. They espoused that if these laws were properly understood and obeyed, it could result in the highest development of the race, the highest type of civilization, and the least incidence of illness.

In his quest to conquer this new field of medicine, however, Rush did well-intentioned experimentation on patients often using questionable apparatus.

Believing that mental illness was in part an arterial disease that caused inflammation in the brain, Rush invented a "tranquilizing chair".

Known as the Rush Chair, it was used for most of the nineteenth century in almost every mental hospital in the country. The chair was intended to reduce blood flow to the brain by binding the patient's hands and limbs, while another apparatus was put over the head to deprive them of sight and sound. Unfortunately, the chair was often used as a restraining device to settle unruly patients.

Dr. Rush was also an advocate of purgation or blood letting, believing that most diseases traveled through the blood stream. He readily made use of homeopathic remedies employed by those outside the stream of accepted medical practice.

While some of his treatments were questionable, Rush proved his basic tenant to be correct, that mental illness was curable. His success rates were promising, even amazing.

In the 1840's the movement got a boost from an unlikely source. This time it was not a doctor or a scientist, but a reformer with the zeal of an evangelist. It took Maine-born Dorothea Dix to bring national attention and action to the plight of the mentally ill and stir the conscience of a nation.

Dix was the daughter of a Methodist circuit-riding preacher, but raised in Boston by her grandmother in wealth and privilege. She first became aware of the wretched conditions of the mentally ill while teaching a Sunday school class for women in a Massachusetts jail, where she made a harrowing discovery.

She saw obviously mentally ill inmates, male and female, clumped together with hardened criminals in unheated, sordid and cramped quarters. Some were even in chains.

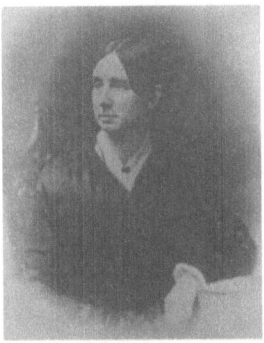

Dorothea Dix was a champion for the care and treatment of the mentally ill. Born in Maine, she worked with her friend Dr. Isaac Ray at enhancing services at the Maine Insane Hospital.

Dix now had a new mission: to comfort the afflicted and afflict the comfortable. Dix used her grandmother's societal influence to get a hearing before the Massachusetts legislature, where she voiced her findings before representatives.

> *I proceed, Gentleman, briefly to call your attention to the present state of insane persons confined within this Commonwealth, in cages, stalls, and pens! Chained, naked, beaten with rods and lashed into obedience.*
>
> *...Some may say these things cannot be remedied, these furious maniacs are not to be raised from these base conditions. I know they are. I could give many examples. One such is a young woman who for years a raging maniac, chained in a cage and whipped to control her acts and words. She was helped by a husband and wife who agreed to take care of her in their home and has slowly recovered her senses. (4)*

Dix took her crusade through most of America and then to Europe. She began to tour other prisons and jails only to make the same discovery and sometimes even worse. Through her efforts, it is estimated that over 123 new psychiatric facilities opened in the United States.

She failed however, in her endeavor to make mental hospitals land grant institutions like the state universities were becoming. In 1848, she appealed to Congress asking that five million acres be set aside to build hospitals, and the remaining land sold to establish an endowment to keep them operating.

In 1854, the bill was approved by both houses, but was vetoed by President Franklin Pierce. In his veto message, Pierce said:

> *If Congress has the power to make provision for the indigent insane, the whole field of public benefice is thrown open to the care and culture of the federal government. I readily acknowledge the duty incumbent on us all to provide for those who in the mysterious order of providence are subject to disease of body or mind, but I cannot find any authority in the Constitution that makes the federal government the great almoner of the public charity throughout the Untied States.*

Dix was undeterred and continued her reform efforts and was instrumental in the growth of the Maine Insane Hospital. The hospital was on its way to being a model for the nation and on the cutting edge of treatment and research.

By the 1950's the Maine Insane Hospital, now known as the Augusta State Hospital, would have been a marvel to its founders. But so would the extent to which mental illness continued to grow its ugly root in the lives of Maine citizens.

CHAPTER FOUR

DIAGNOSIS AND TREATMENT

"I am very sick in mind and in soul"

Constance Fisher, March, 1954

DOCTORS WASTED LITTLE TIME in trying to get to the bottom of the most bizarre case they had ever seen or studied. The first step would be a psychiatric evaluation, given shortly after Mrs. Fisher was admitted to the hospital.

She was first interviewed by Dr. P.W. Lighthart:

> *This patient was interviewed by the writer the evening of her admission. She was in bed, fairly quiet, but showing signs of well-controlled uneasiness. She took the examiner's hand after a while and had the appearance of looking for support. She appeared to be well-reasoned about her name, age, husband, the hospital and referred that something dreadful had happened...*

For the next 30 days Constance was under constant surveillance and put on a suicide watch. She would be visited at intervals by doctors, nurses, and other staff. Her privileges were limited, but she was allowed to go upstairs for an occasional movie.

Carl was there whenever possible, and friends were able to send her gifts and letters.

After the initial battery of psychological testing and interviews, Dr. George A. Sakheim wrote an evaluation summation. In a striking manner, Sakheim stated there was plenty of blame to spread around. He also recognized that it was the disease, not the person, that caused the atrocity.

> *There is little doubt but that this tormented woman deserves our pity and compassion. She seems to be oscillating constantly between realization of the magnitude of her deed and the reflection of defense against the realization of her guilt.*
>
> *It seems to the writer that no useful propose can be served by punishing her for her crime against society as though she were a mentally normal person. It must be difficult enough for her to live with herself without adding to her burden the unnecessary reproaches and the blame and censure of her environment.*
>
> *…It seems to this examiner that there were several warnings of this woman's approaching mental breakdown, in the form of homicidal and suicidal attempts. That these warnings were not heeded is not her fault, but the fault of the ignorant, indifferent, or irresponsible people who knew her at the time.*
>
> *Mrs. Fisher is a woman of superior intelligence who is suffering from the ravages of schizophrenic psychosis. Because of her high intelligence, rich inner resources, the recent onset of her illness, her capacity for insight and strong desire to be helped, it is the opinion of the examiner that this distraught and unfortunate woman may be helped by psychotherapy towards a better adjustment and the acceptance of the tragic fate of her family and herself.*

Dr. Sleeper added to the diagnosis. He wrote:

> *Peculiarly enough, she does not seem to realize that the acts she has committed were wrong in themselves. She has tried to destroy herself on several occasions but changed her mind after each attempt. She claims that she finally thought it would be wrong to destroy herself and leave the children behind so she thought of ways and means whereby she and the children could go to heaven*

together. She now wishes to be helped so she may go home again and live in happiness with her husband.

Dr. Sleeper would leave no stone left unturned in ruling out any medical condition that might be at the root of her illness. He made sure that as far as medical science could determine, there was nothing wrong with her organically.

He even contacted specialists outside of the hospital. When the results of Mrs. Fishers electroencephalographic recording were found outside the normal range, Sleeper enlisted the services of Dr. Milton Greenblatt of the Boston Psychopathic Hospital at Harvard Medical School.

While acknowledging the irregularities, Dr. Greenblatt responded by saying his findings were inconclusive.

On March 12, 1954, Mrs. Fisher was subjected to one of the most painful diagnostic procedures of the time, the spinal tap.

Dr. Sleeper believed that abnormalities in mood and thought sometimes had a biological trigger. And one of the few tests available was the lumbar puncture, also used to diagnose meningitis and seizure disorders.

A small hollow needle, one to two inches in size, was carefully inserted into Mrs. Fisher's lower back without even a topical analgesic to ease the pain. Two vials of cerebral spinal fluid were then drawn to be evaluated in the lab.

The procedure was not only painful but risky. A botched incision was know to produce migraine scale headaches, trauma to the spinal chord, and on rare occasions, paraplegia.

Once again, the test proved inconclusive.

Other diagnostic procedures showed hints of physical abnormalities. Constance entered the hospital running a small fever and complained of muscle pains in her arms and shoulders.

The summation report of her physical exam read in part:

> *...The possibility of an illness affect to the central nervous system temporarily and periodically occurred to us. The possibility of an infestation with a virus of the encephalitis lethargically type cannot be ruled out entirely. Her sore throat, repeated colds,*

and flu, point in that direction. We also think of the possibility of infestation of ascaris or dogs ascaris...

Most of these parasites have a larval stage. These larvae migrate through the lung muscles and also in their migration often end up periodically in a fair amount in the brain. We are therefore highly interested to know if you see any evidence in the chest x-ray which would point to any change, infiltrations or marking, possibly connected with the previously mentioned disease.

Mrs. Fisher was also given the Wechsler Adult Intelligence Scale. Psychologist William Lajousky, Jr., gave the following analysis of the results:

... Expressed in percentile form, this would mean that her I.Q. when compared with a percentile ranking of the I.Q's in the American Population, falls within a range of from the 98th to the 99th percentile. People falling within this range of intellectual functioning are described as having very superior intelligence.

For the first six months of her stay, a court-ordered observation, Mrs. Fisher was not actively treated for her illness. This was due to her impending trial and also because Dr. Sleeper was not exactly sure how to treat this most challenging patient.

While extensive diagnostic procedures continued, Dr. Sleeper was busy calculating a treatment plan. His little black bag was full of procedures that might bring relief and maybe even restoration to one very tormented soul.

And if he ran out of ideas, the school of psychiatric nursing that Sleeper had recently re-established on campus, would be up on the latest research and could contribute some fresh insight.

In the early 1950's, the most promising cure on the horizon was the advent of anti-psychotic drugs like Thorazine and Chlorpromazine. It was hoped that in the development of pharmaceuticals to treat mental illness, a silver bullet would be found. And just as new wonder drugs like Streptomycin were emptying the tuberculosis sanitariums, these new anti-psychotic agents might empty the mental hospitals.

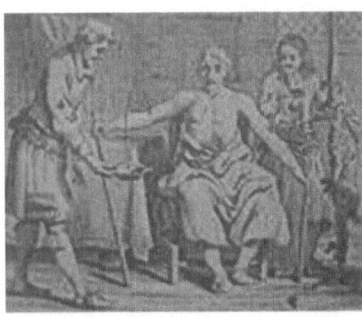

The practice of Bloodletting dates to ancient times. It was thought to be a cure all for illnesses of the body and mind.

Although anti-psychotic medications would prove useful in treatment, they were not benign substances. In some cases, the cure could be worse than the ill. The first generation of anti-psychotic medications produced serious side effects such as kidney failure, diabetes, seizures, and pre-mature death.

And the new field of pharmo-psychology was not without its critics. Were the drugs curative agents, or only effective in suppressing symptoms? Were they being used in hospitals as just another type of restraint? And what would their long-term side effects be?

But at least for now, they could quiet the patient enough that a holistic solution to the problem might be applied.

Another promising treatment option was the various talk therapies which had the plus of rendering no physical side effects. REBT or Rational Emotive Behavior Therapy, was a type of psychotherapy that was short-term, structured, and focused on present situations and conscious choices.

Re-motivation therapy was also proving helpful to many patients. REM focused on the well, healthy, and unwounded aspects of the patient's psyche. They were taught to recognize their strengths and accomplishments, and use them as a springboard to gain health in other areas.

Then there was the staple of most psychiatry of the day, Freudian psychoanalysis, that dealt with childhood traumas, and used dream interpretation and other techniques to look into the workings of the subconscious mind.

Dr. Sheikm felt that talk therapies in particular, would be of great advantage to Mrs. Fisher, an opinion confirmed by Dr. Marquadt. At the least, they would offer her a feeling of support and encouragement. At best, they might provide an understanding of how Mrs. Fisher rationalized the murder of her three children.

Dr. Sleeper also arranged interviews with family members to see if her problems may have stemmed from a childhood trauma or spousal abuse by Carl.

Foster sister Virginia Marcoux said that until the last eight months there had not been even a hint of mental illness. She said that her depression seemed to start right after she finished weaning her baby.

Father in-law Norman Fisher said that you could not have asked for a better mother to the children. Carl said that he and Constance had a happy, fulfilling marriage and that she loved having children, and enjoyed being pregnant.

Revealing, however, was an interview conducted on March 14, 1954, with Ursula Marcoux, Carl and social worker Phyllis Flynn:

> *Mrs. Marcoux is a very talkative individual who expressed a great deal of concern for the patient, stated that it must be God's will that this should have happened. Even though she had just attended the funeral of the three children who were killed, and was discussing a person whom she had brought up since the age of two, she showed remarkably little emotion.*
>
> *Mr. Fisher still seemed to be in a daze and whenever he tried to answer a question worker put to him, Mrs. Marcoux would take over again and give the facts as she saw them... (Carl said) just before her periods patient would become quite depressed and confused and did not seem to know how to do even ordinary routine chores, such as setting the table, sweeping the floor etc.*
>
> *This confusion would occur approximately three or four days before she started her period.*

Dr. Sleeper also used a more subtle avenue for acquiring information. He enlisted the services of Rev. A. J. Lemire, a Catholic priest from the nearby Oblate Center in Augusta, to befriend and council Mrs. Fisher.

In cases like this, when a religious motivation was in play, insights from clergy were considered in-valuable in seeking to understand the motive behind the action. And the Sacrament of Forgiveness and Reconciliation might prove to be more effective in her healing than any drug or treatment.

If all else failed, however, Dr. Sleeper could call upon more radical means.

In a small, well-concealed, room in the Elkin Medical Surgical Building, was a well-fitted operating room used for psycho- surgery, the most controversial tool in treating mental illness at the time.

The notion that literal surgery on the brain might be a way of treating and curing mental illness went back to the 1890's when Freissweixh Golz, removed parts of his dog's temporal lobe and found him to be calmer, less aggressive.

His work was furthered by Antonio Moniz, a medical researcher at the University of Lisbon Medical School. He found that cutting the nerves that run from the frontal cortex to the thalamus in psychotic patients significantly helped some of them.

Moniz devised the first lobotomy procedure by drilling two small holes on either side of the forehead and inserting a surgical knife. The knife was used to sever the prefrontal cortex from the rest of the brain.

Although Moniz had success with the procedure, he advised great caution in using it. He said it should be used as a last resort, in cases where everything else had failed. He was awarded a Nobel prize for his work on lobotomies in 1949.

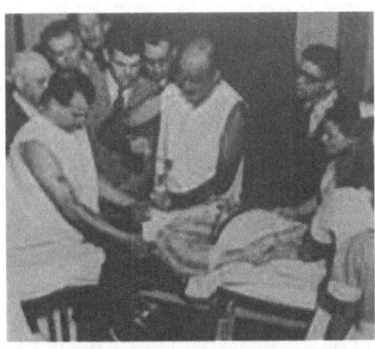

Dr. Walter Freeman performing one of his "ice pick lobotomies."
Dr. Freeman had notable successes and failures.

The lobotomy craze that resulted in almost 20,000 operations in the U.S. between 1939-1951, was popularized by Dr. Walter Freeman.

Freeman is famous for implementing what he called the "ice pick lobotomy."

Freeman devised a procedure in which he inserted an ice pick above each eye of a patient, using only a local anesthetic. He would drive the pick through the thin bone of the eye orbit and a light tap of a mallet would sever the nerves of the frontal cortex. Freeman went from hospital to hospital performing lobotomies assembly line style, causing even seasoned surgeons to faint at the sight.

His work and alleged success reached it's zenith when Joseph Kennedy consulted Dr. Freeman about his daughter Rosemary, who had some behavioral and cognitive difficulties.

One historian wrote:

> *Joe Kennedy began talking to a quack physician from George Washington University named Walter Freeman, who was experimenting with a new form of brain surgery that would come to be known as a pre-frontal lobotomy.*
>
> *...Soon thereafter, Rosemary was wheeled in the operating room. She received a shot of Novocain and when she regained consciousness, her head was on a sandbag. Freeman and his associates drilled a hole in her skull and inserted a sort of spatula into her brain and began digging.*
>
> *They asked her to sing simple songs and perform basic addition and subtracting. As long as she could recite the doggerels and handle the third grade arithmetic, they kept digging.*
>
> *Finally though, Rosemary Kennedy fell silent and the operation was over. And so, for all practical purposes, was Rosemary Kennedy's life. (1)*

Sleeper opted against lobotomy surgery for Mrs. Fisher believing it to be too risky. And given the notoriety of the patient, a public relations disaster for the hospital might ensue if the procedure failed.

The hospital was also equipped with another promising but controversial treatment, electro convulsive therapy or ECT.

With recent refinements in the apparatus and procedure, Dr. Sleeper had reintroduced ECT at the hospital in the late 1940's. It soon became the treatment of choice, and one that Dr. Sleeper had much confidence in. In 1954, the year that Mrs. Fisher was admitted, the hospital treated 382 patients, the vast majority receiving at least some measure of relief.

The drawback was that nobody exactly knew how shocking the brain with electric current actually worked, although history records that electricity has been used in the treatment of mental illness since ancient times.

The first recorded electrical procedure was the Roman physician Largus treating the Roman emperor Tiberius for depression by wrapping an electric eel around his head.

Dr. Sleeper had much more sophisticated equipment to administer the procedure when Constance Fisher became his patient. In the 1950's, the treatment ran a pulse of electric current of about 200 volts for up to 0.5 seconds in order to induce a therapeutic seizure. The seizure would last about 15 seconds, before the patient lapsed into unconsciousness.

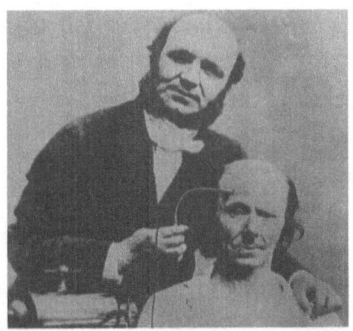

Using electric current to treat mental maladies has been used since antiquity. The Morton Wimshurst Influence Machine was used at the Maine Insane Hospital in the early 1900's.

While treatment options were slowly studied and debated, doctors formulated a diagnosis for Mrs. Fishers' illness. The diagnosis would be important not only in determining her treatment, but also crucial to the insanity defense she would plead, as her day in court was drawing near.

The official diagnosis for Constance Fisher read: **Schizophrenia, paranoid type.**

The diagnosis was shattering to Mrs. Fisher and her family. Schizophrenia is considered to the mind what cancer is to the body. And while one can kill you, the other can make you wish you were dead.

Both have relatively low cure rates. Both seem to come from out of nowhere, dismantling even the strongest and the brightest. Both can go into remission, only to return again with a vengeance.

A schizophrenic is thought by many as a person having multiple or split personalities, which is not the way psychiatry uses the term. It is a disease that causes mood swings, depression, hallucinations, and disconnects from reality.

In June of 1954, Dr. Sleeper reached a decision on what he felt to be the best course of treatment for Constance Fisher. It was a radical approach that offered no guarantee of a cure at a considerable health risk.

The procedure was considered cruel and barbaric by mental health advocates of the day and would be outlawed by the next generation of lawmakers and physicians.

Although studies showed that the treatment met with considerable short term success, over time it left patients grossly obese, caused brain damage, and produced seizure disorders.

And Dr. Sleepers student nurses could have told him that the latest research was showing that those who did find relief often had a relapse.

Starting on August 16, Constance Fisher would begin her first of 26, Insulin Deep Shock therapies.

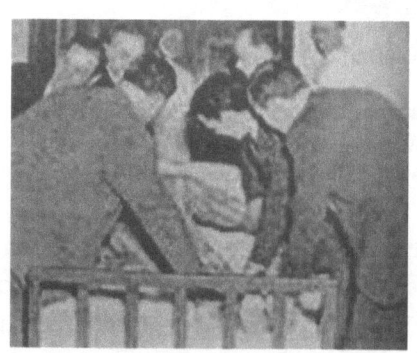 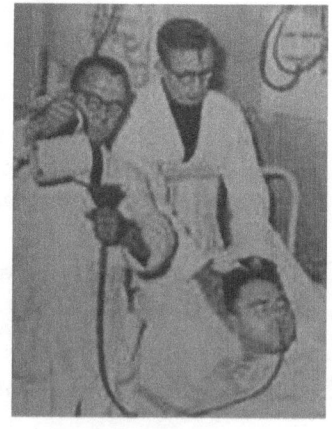

Insulin shock therapy was a treatment of choice in the 1950's for schizophrenia. Presently, it is viewed as a cruel practice that has no reliable evidence of efficacy.

While used infrequently, insulin deep coma therapy was a viable choice in the 1940's and 1950's for those who were considered radically mentally ill. By the late 1940's, it was practiced by most all psychiatric hospitals in America, mostly for the treatment of Schizophrenia.

Its inventor, Dr. Manfred Sakel, claimed an almost 80% recovery rate in the treatment of patients with schizophrenia.

The why was unknown. Sakel explained it as "causing an intensification of the tonus of the parasympathetic end on the autonomic nervous system, by blocking the nerve cell, and by strengthening the anabolic forces, which induces the restoration of the normal function of the nerve cell..." (2)

Perhaps he didn't know either.

Unlike other treatments that would simply mask or quiet symptoms, insulin shock therapy was considered a legitimate attempt to cure the illness. Some psychotherapy was done in the twilight stage between consciousness and coma, but it was believed that the seizures caused by the procedure were themselves therapeutic.

The procedure is dramatically portrayed in the popular film, "A Beautiful Mind," the story of mathematician Dr. John Nash who despite his bizarre delusions and breaks from reality, won a Nobel prize for math in 1994.

A riveting scene in the movie shows Dr. Nash strapped to his gurney as a violent seizure, hard enough to break bones, was induced by the high quantities of insulin he ingested.

For the most part, Mrs. Fisher's insulin shock therapy was unfruitful. It failed to produce any information from her sub conscious recall, and there was no lessening of her anxiety or depression. An unfortunate side effect of the nearly two months of treatment was that Mrs. Fisher gained 30 lbs.

A note attached to her medical chart dated August 27, 1954, however, stated that she went into crisis when an induced seizure turned grand mal and lasted nearly four minutes.

A record given by attendants reveals:

> At 8:00 a.m. Mrs. Fisher was retrieved from her room and wheeled on a gurney into a special room on the third floor of the Stone Building that was set up to receive patients for the procedure.
>
> Breakfast was skipped and she had not eaten since the supper meal.

At 8:30 a.m. attendants began to give her injections of insulin, slowly built up until Mrs. Fisher became near comatose at 200 units of insulin.

At 8:45 a.m. doctors and staff kept track of her vital signs and were ready to write down any information she might reveal during the pre-comatose period.

At 9:00 a.m. she started to perspire profusely and would for the next hour.

At 9:30 a.m. her pupils began to dilate and she went into a stupor followed by twitching of limbs that was first moderate then severe.

At 10:00 a.m. she was in crisis. Her pulse rate had jumped from 68 to 116 and she began convulsions ordinary to grand mal seizure. As a precaution, Mrs. Fisher was strapped to her gurney to prevent injury, with an orderly on standby with a tongue depressor to prevent choking on her tongue, or ready to lay her on her side to prevent choking on her own vomit.

At 10:30 a.m. doctors called in to administer an I.V. of glucose given intravenously to end the coma.

At 11:00 a.m. she was wheeled back into her room and placed in bed.

Ward notes for the next several days reveal that Mrs. Fisher suffered no physical injury from the dangerously extended seizure. For the next four days, she apparently slept off whatever ill effects may have occurred.

A medical record dated September 28, 1954 gave this summation of Mrs. Fisher's insulin shock therapy:

On the 13th this patient was told that she would be placed on Insulin Deep Coma therapy on the 16th. At first she seemed somewhat surprised, but then responded in a rather laparic manner stating that she was glad to learn something is about to be done. She now feels that she is not being neglected and is being given a chance to look for a brighter future...

The writer as well as the psychology department and members of the nursing service are in full attention that now is the time for most alert supervision without any relaxation in the hope that a

lethal exit can be prevented. Carl (her husband) was encouraged
not to visit during the course of her treatment.
　…This patient has up to now received twenty-six insulin
deep shock therapies. To all appearances she is somewhat more
depressed than she was prior to the commencement of the treat-
ment. At no time did she voluntarily give any information nor did
she ever explosively drift into the psychotic reliving of her psychic
trauma experienced during the psychotic acts she committed prior
to her commitment.

It may have been that Constance Fisher's problem was as much
theological as it was physical or psychological. Her improper understanding of Catholic doctrine may have provided enough justification,
or even a motivation, to commit her unconscionable crimes.

The Roman Catholic Church is one of the greatest advocates on
earth for the sanctity of life; in vitro, through life, and end of life. The
Ten Commandments are the cornerstone of Catholic theology, encom-
passing the "thou shalt not kill" edict found in the sixth commandment.

But according to the Catholic Catechism, any baptized child that
dies and is under the age of seven is automatically and instantly transported into heaven.

A popular Catholic funeral eulogy reads:

　…This Faith of ours, this glorious Catholic Faith, has for
centuries boldly proclaimed that an infant who is baptized and
then dies, as our child has, is carried direct to the waiting arms
of God to enjoy the Beatific Vision and live in Paradise Forever.
We as Catholic parents are called by our vocation to strive above
all else to work toward helping our children arrive in Heaven
someday. (3)

Was this a part of Constance Fisher's thought process as she con-
templated killing her children?

Dr. Isaac David was obviously thinking along these lines when he
interviewed Mrs. Fisher on March 25, 1954, about two weeks after she
had drowned the children:

> Q. *I would like to know a little bit about-- you are Catholic aren't you?*
> A. *Yes.*
> Q. *How old has a baby to be before the burden of sin is on them?*
> A. *Seven.*
> Q. *Your oldest was six so there was still time. What was the thought in your mind at the time this happened?*
> A. *I don't know-haven't been thinking too much about it: they told me not to...*

Although Mrs. Fisher had grounds to believe that she had done her children a service by delivering them from an evil world and transferring them into a blissful one, the determination of her own fate was a little more nebulous.

Catholic theology holds for a trinity in the after-life. The elect, or saints, gain immediate entrance to paradise as well as baptized children. The wicked and Godless are incarcerated in a place of punishment called hell. Between the two extremes is Purgatory, a place for those not good enough for heaven or bad enough for hell.

Purgatory is the place where one can atone for past sins and where a soul can work out its salvation and eventually enter heaven.

Perhaps this is why Mrs. Fisher chose as her mode of death the burning, wretching outcome of swallowing the poison shampoo. This might count towards the purgation process and hasten the time when she could be reunited with her children in heaven.

Then, there was the question of the voice that had the ultimate say and responsibility for the tragedy.

A quick visit with Father Holihan would have assured her that any voice commanding her to kill her children was not the voice of the God they served.

He would have told her that killing her children ran against the grain of everything she had learned as a Catholic. Had not Christ Himself spoken of the outcome of those who would injure a child, the most innocent in the human family?

And whoever causes one of these little ones (children) to stum-

ble it would be better for them to have a millstone tied around their neck and be drown in the depth of the sea. (4)

An interview with Mrs. Fisher, by Dr. Sleeper, dated March 25, 1954, is startling:

> Q. *We will be as brief as we can, Mrs. Fisher. May I ask this question? If you will be kind enough, for the purpose of the record, to try and remember. We won't bring this up again—just what the precipitating factor that brought you to do away with your children?*
> A. *It seemed that I was so mixed up and the world was so mixed up, I would never be able to bring them up right.*
> Q. *Was anybody talking to you and telling you what to do?*
> A. *That's what I was trying to remember. It seemed like I did hear a voice, but most of the time it seemed like a presence.*
> Q. *Whose voice was it and whose presence?*
> A. *I was trying to find out if it was God or the devil.*
> Q. *You thought it was God at the time?*
> A. *Sometimes I did. I did not know if it was God or not.*
> Q. *How do you feel about it now?*
> A. *I have been trying to think that it was God's will and somehow it will all work out for the better.*
> Q. *You think you acted in response to God's command?*
> A. *Yes.*
> Q. *Did this voice seem very near?*
> A. *Yes, it did.*
> Q. *At the time you thought it was God's voice?*
> A. *Yes, it seemed to feel as though something was pushing down on me and pushing me toward something.*
> Q. *You heard a voice commanding you to kill your children?*
> A. *That's what I was trying to remember. It seemed like I did hear a voice, but most of the time it seemed like a presence.*

To the doctors treating her, the voice was nothing more than a psychotic delusion, an auditory hallucination. But what if the voice Constance Fisher heard was not imagined after all? What if it was real...?

69

CHAPTER FIVE

THE DEVIL MADE ME DO IT

"God's plan made a hopeful beginning, But man spoiled his chance by sinning. We trust that the story will end in God's glory, but at the present the other side's winning."

Poem by Constance Fisher, June 1955.

"THE DEVIL MADE ME do it..."

So exclaimed comedian Flip Wilson on his popular variety show airing on NBC in the 1970's. The reference was, of course, to the devil being responsible for Wilson's irreverent satire and the audience loved it.

But maybe it is not so funny after all. Maybe there is substance to the glib, foolish sounding phrase. Maybe the heinous acts of a Hitler, Stalin, Manson, or Son of Sam serial killer David Berkowitz, were inspired by a force greater than a depraved human personality.

Perhaps it was the devil motivating the inhuman acts of serial killer, sadist, cannibal, and pedophile, Albert Fish, responsible for over 16 murders and molesting over 400 children in a 14-year period. Fish was finally caught after the murder of Grace Budd in 1934, after he had molested, killed, dismembered, and eaten his innocent victim.

Under this supposition, man's inhumanity to his fellow man takes on another dimension... he has some help.

In the Fisher case, the possibility of a demonic influence was one option never considered. Perhaps at the time, such a notion was thought to be in the area of superstition and ignorance. But times have changed.

In this sophisticated world of the 21st century, a recent poll reveals that 92 % of Americans believe in God and 71% of Americans believe in a real personage called the devil, who has myriads of helpers at his beck and call.

Outside of the United States, the vast majority of this planet's inhabitants have no problem believing in spiritual entities that exert a substantial control over the affairs of mankind.

Unseen beings who influence everything from the weather, to political events, to unrest among the races and nations.

And there are paranormal societies in every country who investigate psychic or "other world" phenomenon. Seemingly every town has it's haunted house with reports of apparitions, moving furniture, and voices.

This universal belief in the paranormal is not only manifested in the evolution of the world's great religions, but also in the dark side of spiritual power. Devil and demon worship has been practiced for millennia. And presently, practitioners of the occult and black magic arts are at an all-time high.

Demonic entities are thought to indwell houses and animals, but manifest their highest expression through human beings. Their intent is to deceive, kill and destroy. Their influence is most pervasive when undetected and ignored.

This cosmology is gaining traction in a world that seems out of control and without human solution. It makes some sense out of tragedy, and answers the question of why bad things happen to good people. And science, once wanting to rid the world of such superstition, is now moving to the forefront to help try to explain it.

William James, the father of modern psychology, was himself a believer in the paranormal. The concept that a tormented person's behavior was caused by a demon spirit would not have been beyond the pale for James.

James was educated at Harvard, where he spent most of his academic life. He would, on occasion, challenge his contemporaries not to let a narrow mind prevent an honest appraisal of psychic phenomena.

He found their biggest challenge was not in believing; it was in not wanting to believe, or being afraid to believe.

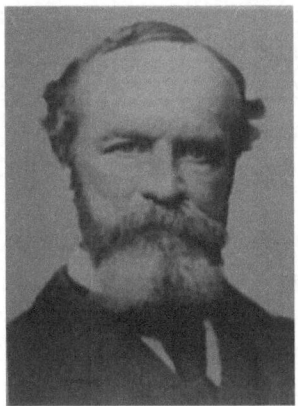

William James, the founder of modern psychiatry, spent much of his academic career in the study of supernatural phenomena. His conclusion was that of the theologians: we are not alone on this planet.

Unfortunately, the work of paranormals and exorcists has seldom found its way to an academic venue. In 2002, however, William D. Tatum took a look at the inhuman acts of several of the 20th century's most sensational serial killers, and wrote the book, "Multiple Murders and Demonic Possession."

Professor Jordan Aumann states the authors thesis in the introduction to the book:

> *The book is the result of many years of investigation and it deserves serious consideration on the part of psychiatrists, judges, and lawyers. He (Tatum) has presented a very weighty argument in support of his thesis, namely that at least some of the serial killers have acted under the influence of a demonic power.*

Malachi Martin writes,

> *....In this idea there is the germ of what Tatum calls forensic theology, namely, in certain cases... the presence among human*

beings of non-human power could in certain cases be the only adequate explanation of the aberrant behavior of such criminals.

The book touches upon the exorcism of Karen Kingston, who at age
seven watched the brutal murder of her father at the hand of her mother.
By age 13, Kingston had turned into a virtual animal, and was placed
in a home for the mentally challenged.

Tatum gives an account of her exorcism conducted by Rev. Richard Rogers. It is a conversation with a demon host called Prudence who
speaks in a mans voice through the lips of the 13-year-old girl:

Prudence:	*Prudence is my name-Karen Kingston's soul is my game.*
Rev. Rogers:	*Is it true that you are a demon of sickness?*
Prudence:	*You will have to guess that, but listen carefully, I'm going to give you a clue.*
Rev. Rogers:	*A clue?*
Prudence:	*(Began reciting a poem)*

Prudence is my name
Karen Kingston is my game
I'm known widely for my fame
For I make people brainless and lame!
So preacher man watch out
I have power you know nothing about
Get in my way, I'll give you a clout
Right on the tip of your long pointed snout!

Rev. Rogers:	*You are required to answer me!*
Prudence:	*Lots of trouble, I cause lots of trouble. You have partial Parkinson's Disease!*
Rev. Jones:	*You are a liar!*
Prudence:	*Yes, I know, but it's all part of the game.*
Rev. Rogers:	*The game? What game?*
Prudence:	*Oh, just the game.*
Rev. Jones:	*You must in Jesus name, on His blood, tell me what game.*
Prudence:	*It's all planned out. We have a planned strat-egy. We know exactly what we are trying to*

accomplish. For instance, we are in almost com-
plete control of this community. We want only
to gain control of the churches. And I'll say this:
you can believe me, we've already taken almost
complete control of the world. You think this
stinking town is any exception, preacher man...

Perhaps the foremost authority on demonology in the 20th century was King's College educated, and Cambridge University professor, Derek Prince. At one time an agnostic, Prince had a spiritual conversion while serving in the British Army in WWII.

He left his position at the university to become an ordained minister. In the late 1960's, while serving as a pastor in a church in Seattle, he had his first face to face encounter with a demon who had possessed and tormented a young housewife. He would spend the next 40 years of his life writing on the subject and performing exorcisms. (1)

In his writings, Prince states that there can be degrees of demonic activity ranging from oppression to possession, when a person is taken over and controlled by a demon spirit. Prince teaches that sprits always have an entry point which can be caused by rejection, participating in occult practices or various forms of sexual immorality. Voice commands to perform an evil deed are common in both demonic oppression and possession.

Prince estimates from the Gospel accounts that over a third of the ministry of Christ involved people He freed from the power of demons.

In the Gospel of Luke is one such account:

When He got out of the boat, immediately a man from the
tombs with an unclean spirit met Him and he had his dwelling
among the tombs. And no one was able to bind him anymore,
even with a chain. Because he had often been bound with shack-
les and chains and the chains had been torn apart by him and
the shackles broken in pieces. None was strong enough to subdue
him.

Constantly, night and day, he was screaming among the
tombs and in the mountains and gashing himself with stones.
Seeing Jesus from a distance he ran up and bowed before Him....

For He had been saying 'come out of the man you unclean spirit' and He was asking him 'what is your name?' And he said to Him,' my name is legion for we are many.'

And he began to implore earnestly not to send them out of the country. Now there were a group of swine feeding nearby on the mountain. The demons implored Him saying 'send us into the swine so that we may enter them...'

They came to Jesus and observed the man who had been demon possessed sitting clothed and in his right mind, the very man who had the legion, and they became frightened. (2)

The story is reminiscent of one found in the superintendent's report for the year of 1840, at the Maine Insane Hospital. Superintendent, Cyrus Knapp, made the following observation of a patient admitted that year:

No. 2 is a man aged 56 of a giant like frame, and immense muscular power-we brought to the Hospital raving and roaring like a lion, and perfectly demoniac in his appearance.

He threatened to lay the Hospital in ruins and destroy every one that came in his way should the least effort be made to interrupt his career. As he passed into the gallery the inmates seemed to shrink back with amazement and terror...

He has been insane a long time and served an apprenticeship of several years at the business of clanking chains in prisons and dungeons.

But there was no Derek Prince at the Augusta State Hospital or any one else to presume that Mrs. Fisher might have had a spiritual problem. A full four years after the murders she still had a sharp, chilling, recollection of the voice and presence that pushed her to act.

Interview with Dr Sleeper June 1958:

Q. Just what did God tell you, how did He command you to kill the children, did he tell you how?

A. Yes, it seemed like that last day before, it seemed like my own idea. I couldn't go through with it. It seemed like that day it was just as if, I don't know, someone took control of me. I was praying to God, either tell me or show me what to do. It didn't seem like it was me that was thinking or doing things at all. You know the day before I have been fighting it off all day. I was awfully nervous, the day before was Sunday and my husband had just gotten a part time job and he worked that Saturday and Sunday. I was fighting it off. I was going to tell him when he came home, but he looked so tired and worried when he came home I didn't want to bother him. The next morning when he went to work I was looking out the window, I almost called him back, but I didn't…that day I didn't seem nervous or anything. When that idea got hold of me I was calm. I just went ahead. It didn't seem as if it was me at all, seemed as if I was an on-looker, looking at a movie, but I wasn't in it.

And again, almost a decade later:

I did what I did because God told me to do it: He said that my children should not live to be more than eight.

It is said that the eyes are a window to the soul. The Fishers' former neighbor, Harold Wilson, remembers the strange, eerie look in Mrs. Fisher's eyes.

Her eyes, there was something about her eyes, they didn't look right. I would see her in town, at the grocery store, she would be with Carl. She did not know me but I knew who she was. Those eyes, she had that look about her, cold and black. It gave you the feeling that you could trust her as far as you could throw her.

Even after almost 50 years, it's a wonder I still don't see them in my sleep…

A psychiatrist familiar with the Fisher case said in 1995:

It's a terrible mystery trying to understand how it happened. She never appeared grossly psychotic. She had no delusions, and she was always a very, very pleasant person. She had a very close family, her husband was devoted to her and she was well liked by the staff.

> *She exhibited no clear signs of mental illness, the two inci-*
> *dents were aberrations and she might have been in a disassociate*
> *state, one that is akin to post-traumatic stress disorder. But that*
> *implies some kind of traumatic event in her early years, but there*
> *was never any record of it.*

As surreal as it may sound, perhaps the devil did indeed make her do it.

CHAPTER SIX

IN HER OWN WORDS

"We will find happiness again someday, I feel certain that you don't really know or appreciate happiness until you have been through the deepest sorrow."

Constance Fisher to her husband, May, 1954

PERHAPS THERE IS NO better way to unravel the tragedy of Constance Fisher than to use her own words. It is a strategy that helps eliminate biases, conjecture, and fading recollections.

It gives the opportunity for those so inclined to conduct their own psychological autopsy.

What follows are portions of interviews, letters, and ward notes from her hospital stay of 1954-1959.

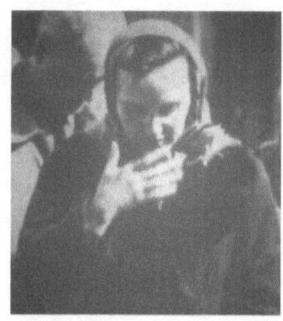

Perhaps there was no one more mystified by the tragedy than Constance Fisher herself. This image was taken shortly after her arraignment and on her way to the Augusta State Hospital in 1954.

Admittance interview with Dr Lighthart:

...I know they are dead. I wish they were still alive. I feel sorry for them, I do feel bad about it, don't misunderstand me. I know that it was not wrong, but they were so young. I wish I had my children back. Do you think I can get more children again now?

Q. Would you kill yourself if you had the opportunity now?

A. No, but I want to be back with my husband and I would like to have other children if I cannot have these back. What am I to do when I get better, do you think I can get better?

The writer answered that we would do whatever we could to help her at this time. Again she squeezed the writer's hand and smiled happily, a smile filled with child-like hope and confidence. She finally stated, "I hope you will be able to help me."

Admittance interview with Dr. Sleeper:

Q. We will be as brief as we can, Mrs. Fisher. May I ask this question? If you will be kind enough, for the purpose of the record, to try and remember. We won't bring this up again- just what was the precipitating factor that brought you to do away with your children?

A. It seemed that I was so mixed up and the world was so mixed up, I would never be able to bring them up right.

Q. *What about the gun you took from your father?*

A. *I knew he had it and I swiped it while I was over at his house. I took it home with the shells, but I could not kill myself, because I was too worried what would happen to the children when I was gone. When I came out of the spell the first thing I did was to bring back the gun and put it where I got it from…*

When she referred to what happened yesterday tears came in her eyes and when asked to tell exactly what happened she first cried for about a minute and then got herself together. She said:

"This time I found the solution. God told me how to do it, I would send my children to heaven and I would not have to worry about them anymore and I could kill myself. I found a bottle of poison and that was what I took, but it did not work…

Q. *What was in the bottle?*

A. *It was a very poisonous shampoo. It was on the label that it was so poisonous that after you use it you should clean your hands carefully even brush to get it from under the nails, but it must be exaggerated because it did not work.*

Q. *You mean it did not kill you?*

A. *Yes. Yesterday morning when I knew therefore how to do it, I filled the tub with water and at 11:30 I took the first one and the second I took at 12:30 I did not think that they understood what was happening and anyway it was for their own good. The oldest one I had to wait until he came out of school at 3:30 and I did the same thing… You know this is all like a bad nightmare, when I wake I hope that it did not happen, but I am afraid it is all true.*

Interview with Dr. Francis Sleeper on her childhood:

Q. *Let's go back to your childhood. Did you have a happy child-hood Mrs Fisher?*

A. *About average, I guess.*

Q. *That isn't what you said when you first came here.*

A. *At the time I thought I wasn't treated right in a lot of ways.*

Q. *Is that story fact or what you just said?*

A. *Well, at that time I really felt that we didn't have a lot of advantages that a lot of our friends had.*

Q. *You are talking about when you were a little girl now?*

A. *Yes.*

Q. *Mrs. Fisher, what was the first outstanding event in your life when you found that you were being put upon?*

A. *That must have been right around three years old. That was when I was living down on the farm with my grandfather and the woman who brought me up, the one I called my mother, and I have since found out that she is really my mother, they visited down there. She married a widower with two children and they lived down there and I was playing with the little boy. He was in the swing and he fell off and they said that I pushed him and they blamed me unjustly.*

Q. *What else happened as you were growing up that made you feel people were against you?*

A. *I felt that my mother and father were against me.*

Interview with Dr. Sleeper on the onset of her illness:

Q. *Do you think you are sane?*

A. *I don't think I am crazy, but once I get these spells I don't know what to do. When I get these spells I can't seem to think for myself. If people tell me I go ahead and do what they tell me…I feel if I could get over these spells I could get along all right. The first thing I would like to have is some little children.*

Q. *Do you recall what happened that day that you got in trouble?*

A. *Yes, I have been trying to get around to writing it down.*

Q. *You don't have to write it, my secretary will write it down, now you tell me.*

A. *The last depression spell started on Wednesday before Ash Wednesday.*

Q. *What were you depressed about?*

A. *Well, I call them depression spells. They started back a little before Christmas. It was just that I had been worrying about money, this and that, my health had not been feeling good for some time. I was worrying all the time. Then I started having these severe depression spells. When I had those spells all I thought of was killing all of us.*

Q. *What is depression to you?*

A. *I don't know, just completely shattered, I couldn't think at all. I thought I had lost my mind. I thought they would bring me here. I didn't know who would bring up the children. I thought rather than trust in the mercy of people, I would trust in the mercy of God…I thought that if we all die together God would give us a chance to start over, because we didn't know the mistakes we had made.*

Q. *How were you going about committing suicide?*

A. *I didn't let myself start thinking about it.*

Q. *But you thought about it?*

A. *Yes.*

Q. *To the extent of how to do it?*

A. *I had three ideas in mind.*

Q. *What were they?*

A. *Hanging, taking a lot of pills, stabbing myself with a kitting needle or clothes hook opened up. The first week I was here the nurses were so nice to me I didn't want to cause them any trouble. If I really got the idea I know a lot of ways I could do it…*

Q. *But you don't feel that way anymore?*

A. *Sometimes I still feel that way. You know at that time I didn't think I would get better. I didn't want anyone else to bring them up. I seem to feel I am getting better now. If the doctors had put me in here in the first place it never would have happened.*

Interview with Dr. George Sakheim after Personality Profile Test:

The patient was cheerful, pleasant and showed no signs of grief, sorrow or noticeable anxiety. She smiled frequently, showed obvious interest in the tests and responded eagerly to praise…there is something innocent, naive and child-like about her manner.

She said that as far as she is able to understand it, her motive in killing her children was a desire for punishment or a desire to escape from responsibility. She said, "the responsibility was too much. I wanted someone to baby me and love me. I have often had a desire to escape into the woods and take the children along with me. I wanted them to escape from all the evil influences in this topsy turvey world…I don't feel I did anything wrong. I miss them awful, but that's part of my punishment. But when I think of them I feel at peace. My last baby was a girl and I always wanted a girl- I nursed her. This brought out all my motherly instinct. I wanted to give her everything. I worried more about her than about the other children. I saw her as myself and I wanted to give her everything I didn't have as a child. I know that self destruction was at the root of it. I kept fighting it off. When I took that poison I thought I was going to suffer a horrible punishment for what I had done. I thought it was going to burn up all my insides.

When I was over one of my spells, I was really high. I sang, danced, and felt full of pep. I would have two weeks of spells and blues and then for two weeks be real high. The spells made me feel as though something was pushing down on me and pushing me toward something."

She mentioned that, after the last testing session, when she returned to the ward, she heard a voice saying loud and clear, "Wait." The voice repeated this word several times in succession. It seemed to come from outside of her and above her. She did not think it was a human voice, but she associated the voice with God. When asked how she felt when she heard it, she said, "I got a little scared. I had a funny feeling."

She wanted to know whether she should accept the blame for what she had done. This again was a very difficult question to answer but the psychologist said that of course, from the point of view of society, it was true that she had killed her children and that society would consider her guilty, but that since this happened in consequence of a mental illness she should not blame herself too much for what she had done.

At this point the patient broke down and sobbed bitterly and said that sometime before the tragic events occurred, she had a feeling that something dreadful was going to happen to her and that she wanted so much to talk to her husband and tell him to bring her down to the state hospital, but she could not bring herself to talk to him.

Interview with Dr. Sleeper on why she killed her children:

Q. *At the time this thing actually happened, what really happened, what precipitated the actual action you took?*

A. *I felt sooner or later the doctor would send me down here (Augusta State Hospital) and I felt there wasn't anyone I trusted to bring my children up as I wanted them to be brought up. I took the pills.*

Q. *You took those pills sometime before the children died?*

A. *Yes, but I was thinking of that at that time. I still had an urge. I wanted to do away with myself before I went down there. The first thing I thought of was doing away with myself. I figured I couldn't do anything right, then I started worrying about the children.*

Q. *How do you feel about it now?*

A. *I realize I was very sick. I remember saying at that time, "I am very sick in mind and soul." I didn't know who to ask. When I went to the doctors they didn't seem to, either they didn't want to help me or couldn't help me. I was worrying all the time. I worried about what effect my illness would have on the children. That made me go to pieces completely, up until that time I was blaming my husband's drinking and this and that. The last time I went to the doctor he said, "You brought it on yourself." That is what started to turn me against myself. Then I started having these severe depression spells. When I had these spells all I thought of was killing all of us.*

Q. *Tell me just exactly how you felt in the depression spell?*

A. *Gee, I don't know, when it first started, as I look back on it now I can see my nerves were going for the last couple of years. I didn't know it then.*

Q. *How did your nerves seem to be going?*

A. *Well, I started out being very irritable with the dog. He got on my nerves so that we had to get rid of him. Then we got another dog and cat and we had to get rid of them.*

Q. *How did you get rid of them?*

A. *My husband shot them I guess. Then I started this worry. I never used to be much of a worrier, but bills got piled up, I hadn't been feeling good for quite a while, started worrying all the time. We seemed to get deeper in the hole and not get anywhere. Bills kept piling up, then we have been trying to buy a house. If he had only given me a good house. I didn't want any nice clothes, all I wanted was a house so I could bring the children up right. I didn't do too bad, they were healthy and smart and everything. I was worrying for nothing of course as I look back on it now...*

Q. What made you think you might be losing your mind?

A. When I had those first depression spells, I couldn't think at all. Couldn't' think of anything. Didn't know what to get for groceries or feed the children. I would stand there a half hour and couldn't make a decision. Then I would grab the nearest thing to me. I couldn't decide what clothes to wear, I would just grab the nearest thing to me and put it on.

Q. Any one in your family ever have any trouble with their minds?

A. No. Not that I know of.

Q. You told Dr. Chasse you thought you were losing your mind?

A. I didn't talk to him very much. My husband thought it was funny. I was awful scared after that time I had tied a nylon stocking around the baby's neck, early in January, I think. I was awfully scared. I called my husband. I didn't know what to do. I left everything up to him. I was scared to go to a doctor. He seemed to think everything would be all right if we moved. My husband did all the moving. I couldn't think at all. I was completely shattered. The children were fighting, and the baby would cry and I would just stand there and cry myself. I didn't know what to do. When I came out of the depression spell I thought that I was all right, but I can see now I was too high, rushing around doing two or three things at once. I couldn't sit down. I thought I was relaxing but my husband would say 'why do you sit on the edge of your chair?' I would think of something to do and I couldn't relax at all. I felt just like a spring wound up tight. When I let go I would go all to pieces...

When I get these depression spells I seem to wake up that way in the morning. It takes all my will power to move, just get out of bed. It takes every ounce of will power just to keep myself going.

Q. Feel as if you are in a daze?

A. Yes, quite, quite dopey, can't think or concentrate to write a letter it would take half an hour to think of a few little things to say.

Interview with Dr. Sleeper on the Voice :

Q. Had you had any strange experience at that time, hallucinations?

A. Yes, down at camp I heard voices.

Q. Whose?

A. I don't know.

Q. What did it say to you?

A. I don't remember exactly, something about, "Only way, you got to do that"

Q. What did that mean to you?

A. Do away with all of us.

Q. Had you ever heard that before?

A. No.

Q. Heard it since?

A. Just once since I came here as I told you.

Q. When?

A. Within the first two weeks, just said, "Wait"

Q. Same voice?

A. Yes, it wasn't distinct.

Q. Was it the voice of a man or a woman?

A. I associated it with a man's voice.

Q Your husband's?

A. No.

Q. God?

A. Yes. God or the devil. I was going to speak with the priest. I had the last spell on Ash Wednesday, and I decided it was God's voice.

Q. When did you hear voices?

A. Only once since I came in here.

Q. When was that?

A. Two or three weeks after coming here, in the large dining room.

Q. What did they say?

A. I just heard voices saying "Wait, wait."

Q. What did that mean?

A. It meant don't do anything rash.

Q. What were you thinking about just before that?

A. That everything was utterly hopeless except suicide.

Q. Was anybody talking to you and telling you what to do?

A. That is what I was trying to remember. It seemed like I did hear a voice, but most of the time it seemed like a presence.

Q. Whose voice was it and whose presence?

A. I was trying to find out if it was God or the devil.

Q. You thought it was God at the time?

A. Sometimes I did. I didn't know if it was God or not.

Q. How do you feel about it now?

A. I have been trying to think that it was God's will and somehow it will all work out for the better.

Q. You think you acted in response to God's command?

A. Yes.

Q. What did the voice say just before you committed the act?

A. I have been trying to think. I would have to stop and really concentrate. I haven't thought about that lately. Said something like, 'you have got to do it,' something like that. The day before voices had been telling me what to do it with, ..I said, I just can't' I haven't got the strength. On the day of the tragedy they said, 'you have got to do it,' and something about being a coward, it's the only way. I think mostly, "you have got to do it." Even then I don't think I would have gone through with it except I started out to give Danny a bath. He said, "I wish I could die in the water." I thought that must be God telling him to say that. Why would he say something like that? Why did he?

Q. When your oldest child came home from school did he know what had happened?

A. No. I started out to do it to the baby in the morning. I couldn't. It was only when Danny said that that it made me go off.

Q. Did your boy come home late from school?

A. Yes.

Q. Do you think he was happy when he left your home?

A. Yes. They were all happy, especially that day. That is why I don't know now why I could think that way.

Q. Did you have to use a lot of force with him?

A. Quite.

Q. Did he see any of the other children?

A. No.

Q. You took something didn't you?

A Yes.

Q. What did you take?

A. Poisoned shampoo.

Q. What make was it?

A. I had to get it on prescription. I thought it was deadly poison. It said on the bottle after using to wash your hands and scalp and dig under fingernails. I thought I was going to die a very painful death, suffer the pain of killing the children, take care of part of the pain in Purgatory.

Interview with Dr. Marquardt on her future:

Q. Since you have been here you wrote your doctors that you are going to plead sane, that you consider yourself sane.

A. When did I write that? I can reason now. Of course, still when I have those depressions, well when I had the last depression I could still reason. I knew it would be wrong to do away with myself, then I wouldn't do it because I knew it was wrong. Before then it didn't seem it. I don't remember writing that to my doctors.

Q. Did you tell anybody that you were gong to plead sanity and take the punishment?

A. When I was first here I talked to Dr. Sakheim, I told him I would take whatever they gave me, if they sent me to jail I would accept it. I want to get better. I feel I am getting better.

Q. So you feel that you were ill and still are?

A. Some, yes. I owe a great debt to society. I can pay it better by getting better than by serving it out in jail. I would like to try to do something to help other people. I would like to have more children, bring them up to be good citizens. I feel that I have done a great injustice by doing away with my children, they were very smart.

89

*Q. How would you try to overcome further excitements and de-
pressions, suicidal and homicidal tendencies?*
A. I don't think I would have any more of those…

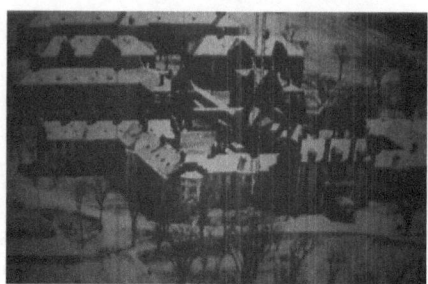

Ariel view of the Augusta State Hospital, winter 1955.
It was from her room in Middle Tyson, (center section) that these
letters were written. The letters were opened and read without Mrs.
Fishers knowledge or permission. Does the end justify the means?

Hospital Letters

To her husband:

Carl,

> *How are you darling?*
> *Please, please write to me as often as you can every night if
> you can and tell me everything you have done all day.*
> *Please don't hate me. You are all I have left to live for. If I
> don't think you still love me I will want to die. I haven't had those
> spells since I've been here but I feel very numb and hopeless.*
> *Please don't forget me. Get out my picture and put it on your
> bureau. It is in one of the boxes up at your mother's. Send me a
> picture of you. One of our wedding pictures will do if you can't
> find the others. … I went to have a brain wave test yesterday and
> had an I.Q. test. We had a movie upstairs this morning, it was
> pretty good but it depressed me to see some of the patients up there.
> I am trying not to get all worried again and am eating good. I do
> want to get better, I hope they will help me here, if only I had come
> before but you told me not to think of the past so I won't.*

I love you dear, please say you still love me, please don't listen to your mother or anybody talk against me. Please write soon and often.

Your loving wife,
Peggy

Dearest Carl,

I missed you Sunday and Monday, did you go to the Windsor fair? Hope you had a good time. I had a swell day Monday. They had a field day in the morning. I entered the contests, won first prize in the sack race, second prize in the tire rolling and third place in the stilt race, not bad huh?

The prizes were candy bars. In the afternoon they had all kind of booths, throwing darts at balloons, bean bag tossing, knocking over things with balls. I won a lot of candy bars on those too, came home with my pockets loaded and won a necklace playing beano and had three bottles of soda, so all in all, it was a very successful day.

Goodbye for now, I love you.
Peg

Dear Carl,

Well, what happened to you yesterday? I was waiting & waiting but at least my mother came, so I wasn't too badly disappointed, but I was hoping to see you.

Martha came back last night with a whole box of food. Her husband could hardly carry it, we had a nice party.

My mother brought me a nice big May basket full of candy. Gin, Agnes and Billy stayed out in the car but I spoke to them through the window.

Please bring me some pictures of the children, also bathing suit, ball point pen, lanolin plus soap, stationary, poker chips, Ivory soap, lobster roll, tissues, Coca cola.

Bring the school pictures of the boys, they were in the green &

white box that was on my sewing machine and the best proof of the baby's pictures which were in a box in the clothes closet.

Lots and lots of love,
Peg.

Dearest Carl,

The nurse just handed me your letter and said, "here's your daily message." You are writing real nice letters, the spelling is still a little off but it gives me a few little laughs at least.

Well I had a surprise yesterday, they called me out to talk to Dr. Sleeper, who is the head one of the whole hospital. I have heard that he is very smart, he certainly sounded it. He was very nice but of course they brought up questions about what happened so I was quite upset. It made me remember all the things I have been trying so hard to forget. I was quite shaky for a long time afterward, but this morning I am calming down again.

The sun is shining very bright here this morning but the breeze is rather cool. Dr. Sleeper asked me why I had asked the Drs. about when my trial was coming up and such. I think they look on it as a good sign that I am showing some interest. The first couple of months, I didn't seem to care what happened but now I really want to get better. He also asked why I didn't talk to nurses more. I said I like them very, very, much but I thought they talked about me a lot. I guess I am overly sensitive about being talked about but he said it was their job to discuss the cases and tell each other how I was acting. I hadn't thought of it that way. In fact I told him the only thing that stopped me from doing anything the first week I was here, was the fact that the nurses had all been so nice to me that I didn't want to cause any trouble for them...

When I left Dr. Sleeper, he said keep hoping. I said I'm not just hoping now, I'm really fighting to get better.

Oceans of love with a kiss on every wave.
Peg.

Hello Sweetheart,

Your letter sounded rather lonesome. I hope the sun's coming out today cheered you up a bit. I will most likely be seeing you before you get this letter but I thought I would write anyhow. I've been thinking about you an awful lot, I love you just as much as you love me, I always have, it was just that our lives get so tangled up that our love alone wasn't strong enough to help us. We didn't have the same sort of life in mind, you seemed to be content with just good enough and I wasn't. Oh well, I won't get all messed up in that thinking just now. I can tell it better than I can write.

Well, they moved Martha this morning, we were both sorry but we had sort of been expecting it so we had been talking about it and we were prepared. She will most likely be going home before long anyhow and she says she will visit me when she can. I am sitting in her room writing this letter, as I always do, so they haven't given it to anyone else yet. I asked for the room the other day but they said not yet.

Yes dear, I hope it won't be too long before I can go for a ride with you, we could visit the capitol again, it's just across the river from here. I can see it every day and it makes me think of you and the time we went through it, remember? It was when we were first married wasn't it?

Carl,

I received your letter that you just mailed this morning-real service huh! As always, I was very glad to hear from you. You must have gotten my letter that I wrote last Friday. Your letter was very sweet and encouraging. I love you too, my darling, I am trying so very hard, I have been very low but I am trying very hard not to let myself go. I hope they can help me when they can give me treatments, they seem to help most of the others. I keep trying but I can't seem to do it alone.

I washed the kitchen floor this morning and yesterday. I washed some windows, I also washed some walls and woodwork in the kitchen. I got a letter from Ethel this morning, very nice, I wrote her last week.

Well, another girl just came in and we are having a cup of tea, it tastes good. We got started taking and it's getting late now so I guess I'd better say goodbye.

With all my love,
Peg.

To her foster mother Ursula Marcoux:

Dear Mama,

…The doctors and nurses are all very nice but the hospital is quite over-crowded and the doctors can't give us much time. I do hope they will help me but sometimes I feel that they don't care if any one of us get better or not but I try not to think or feel this way-I try to keep busy that is the only way not to think & worry-but there isn't much to do-just read-later on I guess they let us do more-knitting and sewing and such -they have occupational therapy but I don't know when I can go to that.

I will be so glad when I can see you- if only I could have talked it over with you before maybe all this wouldn't have happened… I have had a brain wave test yesterday-had chest x-rays two days ago-went to the dentist-my teeth are ok. I have talked with two of the doctors so far, Dr. David and Dr. Marquardt. Yesterday I took some I.Q. tests and I am supposed to take some psychological tests tomorrow. I do hope they can and will help me-it is quite depressing to see some of the cases here- we went upstairs and saw a movie this morning-that ward is worse than this one, really pitiful all of them.

Love,
Peggy

Dear Mama,

How are you this lovely spring day? Isn't this weather wonderful? I will be glad when they let me go out, I was hoping you and

Gin might be down yesterday, but I know you must be awfully busy…

You know Mrs. Proulx, Theresa's mother, she is here, just came in yesterday. She doesn't seem too bad just excited and restless.

Carl is changing quite a bit. I guess the doctors gave him quite a talking to. For one thing he isn't really happy with his work so I told him now is the time to try something he likes because if you don't like your work you can't be contented. He likes mechanic work and carpentry so I suggested these but he said he had always thought that he would like fishing so I told him to go ahead & try if he wants.

I don't know if he is still eligible for GI training or not but he can inquire. A guy he works with had a father in law who has a fishing fleet in Rockland so I told him to talk to him about it. I always liked it by the coast and of course I love lobster so I won't mind. That is what soured Mr. Fisher so, working at a job he hated.

I guess when Carl was young his father used to come home crabby and Carl couldn't make a sound or he would get a licking which is where he got all his initiative knocked out of him because he is smart enough. I am trying to encourage and help him all I can. Even now I guess they are trying to tell him what to do, he is quite disgusted. But I told him to just speak his mind and stand up to them. The doctors told him he had to change if he ever wants them to let me go back to him and I told him the same thing myself…

Love,
Peggy

To her sister Jacqueline Chamberlain:

Dear Jackie,

Received your nice little note while we were at dinner. I was very glad to hear from you, Mama says you are getting along fine. I am very glad to hear that. And just when is the approximate date? I believe you already told me once the names you have picked out but I have forgotten so write and tell me again…

Yes, the last month will seem the longest, but try to keep busy and the stork will be here before you know it. I am anxious for you, eager to know if its a boy or a girl;. I know just how you feel. Have you decided on nursing or not? I think you will miss a lot if you don't nurse and will regret it later. It brings you so much closer to your baby, you feel you are doing your duty toward your baby. When we are mothers we have to learn to be unselfish and inconvenience ourselves for the good of our children. God gave woman breasts for that sole function and we should follow His will if we possibly can. I am speaking from experience. I always felt sorry afterwards that I didn't nurse Dickie and Danny. Perhaps all this wouldn't have happened if I had been content from the start...

All my love,
Peggy

To her mother -in- law Alice Fisher:

Dear Alice,

Received your letter this morning and I am very happy to hear that you are getting around quite good now.

Just as I was getting ready to write this letter I received a letter from Carl. The nurse said, "this girl gets a letter every day." I guess they are a little surprised that Carl and you folks have all stood by me so good. You are all wonderful and I'm not forgetting it for one minute.

Thank you from the bottom of my heart for everything you have been and are doing for me.

Love,
Peggy

To Dr. Samson Fisher:

Dear Dr. Fisher,

Just a note to let you know that I am feeling fine and am on the road to recovery-I hope. I heard that you felt very bad over my misfortune and would like to put your mind at ease. My mind is completely cleared up now and I am making the best of things... I have probed my subconscious mind and brought to light all the guilt feeling, fears, and anxieties and have faced and conquered them.... I wish I had learned all this long ago or that the doctors had talked to me more. I could have fought it if I had known what I was fighting but I didn't know. I really thought I was fighting a devil within myself-but it was only my subconscious mind, but I must not start this if only business. It wasn't anyone's fault and I am not blaming anyone. I am trusting in God and I hope that He will forgive me my trespasses as I have always forgiven any trespasses against me.

Peggy Fisher

To Doctor Richard Chasse:

Dear Dr. Chasse,

I thought you might like to hear from me although I imagine Virginia has already told you that I am getting along fine. I haven't had any of the deep depression spells like I had before although sometimes I am up one minute and down the next. I still have a lot of tension but no chest pains like I had before.

I have psychoanalyzed myself and have faced all the problems that were bothering me. For the first time in my life I am truly awake and alive in mind. I know and understand myself which I never did before. I have grown up emotionally, I never had you know, emotionally.

I in no way blame you or anyone else. I expected you and the others to help me when I didn't know enough to help myself but I have learned a lot from this experience . I am trying to derive all the good I can from it in helping others here.

And I also want to help Carl... And I feel that I will have a good many more children someday and will be a much better mother for having been through this experience. But even if they send me to jail, I can take it. I will spend my time praying and someday I'll meet my darling children in heaven. Come and see me sometime when you can.

Peggy

To Dr. Paul Jones:

Dear Dr. Jones,

Perhaps this letter will come as a surprise but a pleasant one I hope. I am getting along fine I thought you might like to know. I have psychoanalyzed myself and I think I have done a good job of it. For the first time in my life I feel really alive and not living in a dream world. I know and understand myself and the reason for my personality. It is a wonderful feeling to know yourself and be at peace with yourself I feel that now I can face anything. If only this had come about sooner with the tragic consequences, but I mustn't dwell on the "if only."

I have heard from Barbara Thomas, a patient of yours who is here, that you were discharged from Thayer. I hope this is not true, and if it is true I hope it is in no way on my account. I have caused enough trouble for everyone without that. I in no way blame your or hold you responsible. I am not blaming anyone.

The first time you talked with me was only 15 minutes and you only had time to get my personal statistics and the second time, I was in one of my high spells and was perfectly normal, so how could you know?

Drop in and see me sometime if you are up this way. The day supervisor on this ward is some relation to you, her name is Mrs. Jones. Well so long and good luck.

Constance Fisher

CHAPTER SEVEN

PICKING UP THE STORY

"The truth is stranger than fiction"

Lord Byron, 1823

IT WAS AMAZING TO me that a story that had twice made national headlines a generation ago, had been all but forgotten by Maine people. There was some recollection of it by older Mainers, but very few remembered any of the details. And they were astounded that it happened twice.

With but a faint recollection myself, I was able to uncover a glimpse of the story from a file at the Maine State Library entitled, "Murders in Maine."

And like most significant discoveries, I happened upon it by chance, or providence, while working on another project.

Accompanied to the library by University of Maine journalism major Michael Shepherd, we were sifting through a stack of brittle and yellowing newspaper cut outs when we reached the March 9, 1954 edition of the Bangor Daily News which told of the first Fisher murders. It was our introduction into the Constance Fisher tragedy, ever pertinent as our government contemplates the overhaul of our nations health care system. It was a story begging to be re-told, that it's lessons might be learned and not repeated.

But Michael and I knew that old newspaper clippings alone would hardly suffice to tell the tale of this tragedy. And we were mindful of the closing window of opportunity to interview any remaining players in a drama that took place nearly half a century ago. We began our research immediately.

Our first effort was to find if there were any surviving kin. A search of the internet revealed that Constance Fisher had died in 1973, and that Carl had died in 1990.

It didn't take long to further narrow the list. Their parents, Norman and Alice Fisher and Warren and Ursula Marcoux, had been dead for many years, as had many of their children.

A newspaper article about Andrea Yates, the Texas woman who had also killed her children by drowning them, gave us our first break.

In the article, two sisters, Virginia Witham and Louise Bowker, had been interviewed and identified as foster sisters of Constance Fisher. An online obituary revealed that Virginia had died in January of 2009, but apparently Louise Bowker was still alive. Michael somehow produced a phone number, and I placed the call.

To my surprise, Louise Bowker politely accepted our request to talk about her sister and the tragedy. And on June 25, Michael and I made our way to Waterville to interview Louise.

But before we did, I first had to satisfy my curiosity. I asked Michael if he wanted to visit the place where the first Fisher murders had taken place, which was within walking distance of the Bowker residence.

He seemed as eager as I to time travel back to the events of March 8, 1954, and view the actual crime scene.

From the newspaper accounts, we determined a physical address, but a lot can change in 56 years.

911 enhancements have changed house numbers. Whole neighborhoods have been leveled by wrecking balls only to rise again as industrial parks or playing fields.

I recalled my grandfathers automobile dealership, Waterville Auto Sales, which once sat just a few blocks away. In 1967, it was plowed into a parking lot by an urban renewal project

And another thought. Who would have wanted to live there after the tragedy anyway? It must have been a very difficult rent to fill, and maybe it never was. Maybe, because of the notoriety of the incident, the building was torn down by the owner.

Also from the newspaper account, we had a physical description of the house. It was a white, two story duplex with a driveway on the east side of the building. Attached to the end of the building was a barn or shed.

Not much to go on, but maybe enough.

Michael and I pulled up to the address and to my delight there was a white, two story duplex with a small barn attached to its north face. The house, although it appeared to be in good condition, was unoccupied.

From the end of the driveway I looked up into the window where Constance Fisher had watched her husband drive off on the morning of March 8, 1954, moments before taking the lives of her children in the bathroom located just to the right. I pondered in silence before hollering out to no one in particular, "Don't do it, Mrs. Fisher, Don't do it!"

Noting the premises was vacant, I traveled up the outside stairway to peek through the windows of the second story flat that was home to the Fishers for the first three months of 1954.

Climbing the stairs I saw a sticker affixed to a bedroom window that at closer examination revealed a child safety advertisement. An amazingly cruel irony, I thought, as I continued up the stairs.

A few steps later, I reached the landing and then the front door that the newspaper article said Carl Fisher had kicked in to gain entry into the apartment on that awful day.

I noted the door, typical of the era with one exception: It was covered with a metal sheathing, the kind a carpenter puts on to salvage a door that is cracked or rotting.

At this point, it was good that Michael was with me. Sometimes a reporters instincts can get the better of him. I noticed that all that prevented me from continuing my investigation from inside the house was a loose dead bolt that I knew I could move with my credit card.

Sensing where I was headed, Michael prophesied the next day's newspaper headline:

**"Writers Caught Breaking and Entering While
Investigating Old Murder Story."**

I looked through the west facing windows and saw the layout of the apartment. I had the general floor plan from the article, and it appeared just as it did almost 60 years before. My mind whirled as I peered in to see the living room area where little Dickie Fisher must have watched Howdy Doody and Carl Fisher had lovingly played with his children.

And then, as I moved to look in the window adjacent to the door, I saw it. The pipe overhead told me I was looking into the bathroom. And there, now in full view, I saw a large, porcelain, white bath tub. I had seen enough...

For some reason, I still wasn't completely satisfied that this was the former Fisher residence. On the way back to the car I noticed two older gentleman, sitting directly across the street having a beer. I told Michael once again I needed to satisfy my curiosity.

After introducing myself, I asked the older gentlemen, who I guessed to be in his late 70's or early 80's, if he remembered the Fisher murders.

"Oh yes," he said, "They happened right across the street," pointing to the building I had just visited. "A very sad story, how could you ever forget it?"

"One more question," I added. "I was just over there and looking in through the window I noticed an old porcelain bath tub. Do you think that it might be the same tub where she drowned the children?"

"It is," he proclaimed matter of factly.

"How do you know?"

"I owned the building."

Michael and I proceeded just up the street to the two-story dwelling where Louise, and her husband, Mark, made their home. Ironically, it was built in the footprint of the old Sirois farm that was home to her grandparents, and Constance until age three. It was later destroyed by fire but rebuilt by Louise.

We found Louise to have a unique gift for making people feel welcome, even those looking to uncover sad memories that would be happier left forgotten. She led us to sit around the kitchen table, and over a glass of lemonade, we made small talk about ourselves. I was interested to find that Louise's father, Warren Marcoux, and my grandfather, Henry Briggs, were rivals in the car business in the Waterville area in the

1950's and 60's. Mr. Marcoux sold Dodge and GMC and my grandfather was the Ford dealer. It must have been a friendly rivalry, however, for Louise produced a picture of all the area dealers gathered around a table for dinner at the Marcoux residence.

It was also of interest to discover that throughout 1950's Carl Fisher drove a Ford, which in all likelihood he bought from my grandfather.

As the pleasantries waned, we got to the heart of the topic. Louise made no bones about the fact that she felt the mental health system had failed her sister and was more than willing to talk about it.

We asked her to start at the beginning, as far back as she knew. She said that Constance, (who she preferred to call Peggy,) had been adopted shortly after birth by her grandparents, Silvier and Rose Sirois. The baby remained with the Sirois family for only a short period until ill health and finally death caused her to be taken in by the Marcoux family as a foster child.

The family eventually consisted of eight children, two from Warren Marcoux's earlier marriage, five of their own, and Peggy.

Despite the difficulty that occurs in blending a family, Louise recalled the Marcoux household as being very loving, caring and stable. Their lives were built around church, family and their summer camp on Snow Pond.

Louise said that Peggy was treated no differently than the other children. As a teenager, she recalled Peggy as being mischievous and in and out of trouble with her parents. She recalled the time that she played hooky from school and made taffy which she hid around the house to eat herself or bribe the other children with.

She remembered that Peggy did not finish her education at Mt. Merici High School, but left after her junior year to marry Carl. They were married in a small ceremony with a reception at the farm. Photos of the wedding and reception had unfortunately perished in the fire that burned down the house.

She recalled Peggy as being a marvelous cook who could knit and make her own clothes, but that house keeping was not her forte. She remembered the first batch of Fisher children, Danny, Deborah, and Dickie, as beautiful children, adored by their parents and grandparents. She recalled Dickie as having green eyes and blonde hair and looking much like his father. Danny was blonde with gray eyes and little Debbie, shy around strangers, had big gray eyes and a narrow face.

She said the children were always well cared for, well dressed, and extremely well behaved. The baby's hair was always in ribbons. Every Sunday, after church, was a big gathering of the extended family at the Marcoux house. Carl and Peggy seemed, from her vantage, like the ideal couple with three beautiful children and much to look forward to.

Louise was not quite a teenager when the first tragedy hit. She recalls attending the funeral service and seeing the small white coffins put in the ground and laid to rest, but little else.

When Peggy was hospitalized at the Augusta State Hospital she would on occasion visit her but not often.

She recalled Carl as a quiet, sweet man, one who loved to garden, hunt and fish. He was tall and thin with a ready smile and a dry sense of humor, she said.

She said he was totally committed to his wife, even under the worst situations imaginable.

"Peggy and Carl lived for each other," she said. "Carl even made the offer to be sterilized if it would help get her out of the hospital."

Louise said that there was no talk of the tragedy among the family and that Constance and Carl never brought it up. Neighbors, church parishioners and even the whole community went out of their way not to ostracize or unfairly treat her.

But in the back of everyone's minds there was always the specter that it might happen again, especially when a new baby arrived about ten months after her release. But then again, they had been assured by the doctors that everything would be okay, and to let nature run its course.

"We really did not give it any thought," Louise said of Carl and Peggy's decision to have another family. "They loved each other and they loved having children, and the doctors said it would be the best thing in the world for her."

After Peggy's release, Louise wondered why Carl never put a telephone in their house, just in case of an emergency. "Maybe it was part of his shielding her from the outside world, I really don't know but the family was always after them to get a phone."

And perhaps another oversight. Why didn't he replace the bathtub with a shower stall?

When the next batch of Fisher children came around, Louise was thrilled to play a part in their lives. She was Aunt Louise to Natalie Rose, Kathleen Louise, and Michael Jon and she loved the role. Once again, she said there was no sign of delinquency as far as parenting went.

"Peggy would have been an excellent home-school mom," she said. The children from a very early age were introduced to drawing, painting, and writing and the older children were reading by the age of three or four."

And the children had every play thing imaginable, maybe too many, Louise thought. Just before the tragedy, Peggy had finished making a Batman outfit for Michael, and a princess outfit for Kathleen.

In the spring of 1966, Louise could see Peggy was struggling again. She observed that trouble began when she stopped nursing her baby, Natalie Rose. "It is strange that both times it was the third child that triggered it, not the first, or the second."

In mid June, Peggy made an appointment with Louise, then a professional hairdresser, to do her hair. Not feeling well, and struggling under the hot, humid weather, Louise had to cancel the appointment. Seven days later, the tragedy occurred.

"I got a call at work that Peggy had killed the children," Louise said. I got in my car and drove to Snow Pond where the family had gathered. I walked out on the dock by myself and looked up to the sky and said, "Why God, why?"

During the years that followed, Louise felt a sense of responsibility for the tragedy. Perhaps if she had she kept the hair appointment she might have detected that disaster was imminent. Or Peggy might have revealed her plan. Or she might have said something to change Peggy's mind. The guilt and regret eventually led her to seek counseling.

Louise recalled the scene of the burial of the children, the three white coffins, the hot summer day, the three other children buried behind the headstone 12 years earlier. She doesn't know how Carl kept his sanity through it all. She recalls the sad, somber mood in the church after the service with no talking or fellowship just a feeling of bewilderment, wondering what went wrong, and "what did we do wrong?"

"If I had to blame a person for the tragedy it would be Kirkpatrick," she said, speaking of Dr. Price Kirkpatrick who was treating Peggy at the time and made the determination that she return home instead of a further stay at Thayer Hospital, or going back to the Augusta State Hospital.

"She did not want to go home, she was afraid to go home, she feared that something dreadful was about to happen, but he sent her back."

Louise Bowker never blamed her sister for the death of her nieces and nephews.

"She was not in her right mind, she was tortured. Her world was so dark that she really believed they would be better off dead.

In her mind, what she did was not an act of selfishness or anger, it was an act of love."

The Andrea Yates filicide resurrected the old and painful memories. After her interview ran in the Waterville Sentinel, Louise tried to reach out to the Yates family but never had a response. Instead, she received hate mail and phone calls concerning her sister and Andrea Yates.

She handled the situation with grace and a dose of stark reality.

"People need to be careful in their judging other people", she said. "A chemical imbalance or a crisis and it could be you."

Bowker said that one afternoon shortly after the Yates tragedy, she was picking up fabric at the house of Judge Donald Marden, son of the judge who issued Constance her freedom in 1959.

She told him that the event was so much like her sisters, to which he commented that even with the advances in psychiatry the doctors still missed it. He further responded,

"My father always felt badly about the last time. He said, "If I had not released her she never would have done it. What was I thinking?"

Louise said she would frequently visit Constance at the Augusta State Hospital, as did her other family members after her commitment in 1966. She commented that with all the noise and crowding, the confusion was enough to make a sane person crazy. She said that Peggy always seemed composed, dressed well, looked well, and kept herself busy with her job of mail and package delivery around the hospital.

Louise recalled that in early 1973, when the court determined that she would never leave the institution, Peggy began to speak of her suicide plans.

"If I am going to spend the rest of my life here, I will drown myself in the river," she told Louise.

Louise mentioned to us the dates of Peggy's two stays at the Augusta State Hospital, 1954-1959 and 1966-1973. I concluded that if she was there that long there must be a record of it, and perhaps evaluations, doctors notes, test results, and who knows what else.

I mentioned to Mike on the way home that the whole project would rise or fall on securing Mrs. Fisher's medical file. They more than anything else, would tell the sad tale of this tragic and tormented life.

Φ Φ Φ Φ Φ Φ Φ Φ Φ Φ Φ Φ Φ Φ Φ Φ Φ Φ

IN OUR DAY THERE is increasing skepticism about our government, federal and state.

Some say it is much too large and inclusive. Others point out that it is ineffective to the point that one department trips over the other causing waste and repetition of services.

Many are sure that it is run by special interest groups, secret organizations, and lobbyists. It is alleged that those in power are primarily concerned with furthering their careers and lining their pockets.

Formerly, I had never bought into such charges. Now, I am not so sure.

The first step in accessing Constance Fisher's medical file was to find out if it still existed, and if so, where it was archived. I knew that many state documents have a destruction schedule, usually 50 years, sometimes less.

Michael and I first inquired of Art Dostie and Anthony Douin at the Maine State Archives who told us that medical records of patients at the Augusta State Hospital going back to the 1840's had all been preserved. They told us that the medical records of Constance Fisher were most likely in storage at the Riverview Psychiatric Center in Augusta.

In 2004, Riverview Psychiatric Center had replaced the 160-year-old facility where Mrs. Fisher had twice been a patient. The old hospital had the capacity to service the needs of 2000 patients with 300 acres to build on if more room was needed. The new facility has about 100 beds, used primarily for short term care. It is, in every way, a shadow of the old hospital.

"With a rising population and corresponding rise in the population of the mentally ill, where on earth are patients now being treated", I asked Mike. This was our first red flag that something in the mental health system was seriously skewed.

Mike filed a brief under the Freedom of Information Act to secure Constance Fisher's medical records that was promptly dismissed. Other attempts to secure her records also failed, or were met by a cold resistance. I was getting the sense that the Fisher file might be implicating of someone or something.

Upon a recommendation, I placed a call to Dan Dodge *, a ranking state medical official. I stated my business and began asking if he knew how I could acquire the records. (1)

Mr. Dodge probed me for information before saying anything. Finally, he acknowledged that he was aware of the Fisher case and said that her records were at Riverview. I assured him that this was a legitimate research project and I already had sources lined up to interview.

He wanted to know their names and I naively gave him the names of Dr. Loring Pratt, Dr. Ulrich Jacobson, and Dr. Nathan Fellows *, all of whom played an actual role in Mrs. Fisher's treatment.

He said, "I want you to know that I am neither for you or against you in your research. It will be hard for you to get much information, but perhaps in the future I might able to help you." Our conversation left me questioning just how helpful he intended to be.

I had an interview with Dr. Pratt the next day so I was content to forget about the call. Dr. Pratt had been most amicable over the phone and seemed eager to talk about the tragedy. With Mike now back at school, I made my way alone to Fairfield where Dr. Pratt, now 91 years of age, lived with his wife Jeanette.

From the expression on Dr. Pratt's face as he greeted me at the door, I knew that something had soured. We exchanged pleasantries before he told me that he had just been informed over the phone that due to doctor/ patient confidentiality laws he could not talk about the case.

"And if you don't mind my asking, who called you, Dr. Pratt?

"Yes, it was Dan Dodge from the ..." Hmmm.

It was a long drive back to Hallowell. In my mind there was something far worse than not getting an interview. Like many Americans who lived through the Nixon years, I have come to disdain obstruction or cover up by people in power.

I had wondered why this official was so coy with me over the phone. And now he was calling people behind my back.

My next attempt at an interview was with Dr. Fellows. I had been told that he was a marvelous doctor that had served at the Augusta State Hospital for nearly half a century. I knew that he would be one of the few, if not the only, physician that had been at the hospital during both of Mrs. Fisher's stays. He was a reporters dream, a gold mine of primary source information!

From a newspaper article about his career, I gained enough information to locate an address and a phone number. I anxiously placed the call.

The tone of his voice after the initial pleasantries told me he was reluctant to talk. If I had probed I am sure I would have found that he too received a phone call from a higher-up.

I asked him if he was familiar with the Fisher case to which he responded, "No, no I don't think so." I said that a colleague of his had recommended that I talk to him and that his perspective would be valuable.

"That is his field of expertise and not mine. I do not care to comment." He finally stated, "I do not remember the case, Constance Fisher, I never knew her."

Overall, my dealings with Maine state government were disconcerting at best. I was constantly encouraged to give up my quest for documents by different state agencies. A meeting with the governor to get his opinion on the case was first excepted, then put on hold, and then declined.

I wandered about the state capitol one day noting that the legislature was in session. What I saw greatly alarmed me and should every citizen and taxpayer. There were pockets of legislators everywhere listening to the pitches of lobbyists.

Our founding fathers would have been appalled to see this bullying of democracy. At best, lobbyists are only "informing" about one side of an issue.

At worst, as in the case of Jack Abramoff, they are using money and influence to secure the votes of our elected officials.

And where were the lobbyists when the Augusta Mental Health Institute was being dismantled and its' occupants cast out to the streets? Who was there to represent the interests of the voiceless and penniless?

I made several attempts to get a tour inside the old Stone Building that the legislature had shut down in 2004. Although it is one of the most historical buildings in the state, it is now mothballed and sits vacant.

I wanted to see the space where the hospital superintendents lived, visit the admissions area, walk through the different wards and treatment areas. I wanted to visit the rooms to get a feel for what it might have been like to be a patient there.

I had a good idea of where Mrs. Fisher's room was, although she had three different ones during her 12 year stay.

I called the Bureau of General Services that had responsibility over the maintenance of the building. I was told that the building had been closed and that no one was allowed in. I found this interesting, for on two different occasions I saw groups going in and touring the premise.

When confronted with the evidence, I was told yes, tours were occasionally given and that I would be put on a waiting list. And wait I did. But after three months of waiting, my patience grew thin and I paid a visit to the state office in Augusta and was seen by a foreman.

I told him that I was having no luck trying to catch a tour of the building, but had seen maintenance people go in at night, which he confirmed. I asked if perhaps I could go in with them on a week night. He said that would not be possible, because there were environmental issues with the building and liabilities.

"What about the tour groups? They seem to pass through alright," I responded. No comment. End of conversation.

Adding to my angst, the following week a paranormal society was given permission to set up their cameras, detectors and recorders in attempt to find spirits and psychic phenomenon on the hospital campus!

I did, however, get the opportunity to see the inside of one building on the campus. It was the old maximum security building, built in 1908 to house the violently criminally insane. It was later converted into office space when the hospital was scaled back, at a hefty sum of tax payer money.

But recently the state had found a better rent, owned, incidentally, by a lobbyist, and had left the building empty.

One day while driving around the hospital complex, I happened upon the building. The heavy glass front door had been broken, and was left wide open. Looking inside, it appeared that people were now squatting there.

It seemed sadly ironic that perhaps some of the same people that had been kicked out years before, might once again be trying to find refuge there.

Φ Φ Φ Φ Φ Φ Φ Φ Φ Φ Φ Φ Φ Φ Φ Φ Φ Φ Φ

O N THE NIGHT OF June 24, I called Dr. Ulrich Jacobsohn, a psychiatrist and former superintendent at the Augusta Mental Health Institute. I was told he could bring to the table an impressive array of scholarship, training and clinical experience. I was not disappointed.

I was, however, a bit taken back by his initial response.

"How are you Bob? I have been waiting for your call," he said as he answered the phone.

"How did you know I would be calling?" I chuckled. "Well, Dan Dodge contacted me and said that you might be calling." Hmmm.

We set up an interview for the next week and on June 29, I made my way to the retirement community where Dr. Jacobsohn makes his home. There I found a robust man, nearing 90, with a very keen mind. He seemed eager to talk about his expertise in life, the study of the human mind and its effect on society when things go wrong.

After exchanging pleasantries, we got right to the point. "Yes, I remember the Fisher case," Dr. Jacobsohn said dryly. He said that while he was acting superintendent at the institution, he became acquainted with the case. He had read her file several times before writing a "psychological autopsy," as he called it, after she committed suicide.

"We were all mystified as to why the tragedies occurred," he said.

He called it one of the most tragic and perplexing cases of any he had encountered in his almost 65 years of psychiatry.

Dr. Jacobsohn said he had spent many hours studying the thick file of doctor's notes, ward notes, tests, and medical evaluations that composed her over 500-page folder.

"We tried hard to understand her and the phenomenon that triggered the tragic events," he said.

I then asked Dr. Jacobsohn the obvious question: what in his opinion was the diagnosis for her illness?

He said that initially he had ruled out post partum depression. He said she did not appear to be grossly psychotic, delusional or schizophrenic. "Rarely, if ever did she manifest signs of mental illness during her stays at the hospital," he said.

Dr. Jacobson believed that at the time of her murders she was in a disassociate state, and was not aware of her actions. His fellow doctor, and friend, Dr. Walter Rohm had come to a similar conclusion. Dr. Rohm had labeled her illness Oneirophrenia, a type of schizophrenia that causes a hallucinatory, dream like state where the victim is often unaware of his or her actions.

Before I left, Dr. Jacobsohn gave me a piece of advice.

"If you want to see her records, try to find a next of kin if there are any still left alive. They cannot deny next of kin a look at any medical records."

I called Mr. Dodge early the next day to see if this was so. He said yes, if there were any records, they could be secured by getting a consent form signed by a next of kin. I asked where I could get such a form and he answered by giving five different phone numbers to call. "And if they don't work, I might be able to give you more," he said.

They didn't work. I spent most of the morning chasing answering machines and talking to people who had no knowledge, or could only pass me on to someone else. I spent a good part of the afternoon following the same course, and waiting for phone messages that were never returned. I quit about 2 pm.

The next day, I took it upon myself to go straight to the source and visit Riverview Psychiatric Center. I went to the administrative desk, requested the form, was given the form and received straightforward instructions on how to fill it out.

I wasted no time in heading to Waterville to get Louise Bowkers approval and signature for a release of the documents.

The next morning I took the signed consent form to Riverview where I met Elaine Wyman, who looked over the paperwork, found it to be in order, and scheduled a time for Louise and I to peruse the medical file of Constance Margaret Fisher.

On July 19, I met Louise in the parking lot of Riverview Psychiatric Center. She was dropped off by her husband Mark who asked me how long we would be. "I have no way of knowing, there are a lot of documents to go through," I said. Give us maybe three hours."

As Louise and I made our way to the hospital lobby, Louise looked over her shoulder at the stately old Stone Building that was twice home to her sister. It had been nearly 40 years since her last visit, just a short time before Constance had committed suicide.

She turned and took a deep breath before entering the lobby. I asked her if she was going to be alright, if she still wanted to go through with it? She gathered herself, straightened upright, and responded, " Yes!"

Once inside, we were given a visitor's pass and escorted through a series of locked doors that required the swipe of a security card to get through.

The feel of the building was more like a prison than a hospital. On the first floor, most of the space was administrative offices. Patients were conspicuously absent. Although modern, the architecture exuded a cold, sterile feeling.

We were then met by Elaine Wyman who led us into the archives section. I looked up at the rows of steel bins that contained the stories of the thousands of patients that had spent time at the hospital since 1840. Could any of those be as sad as that of Constance Fisher, I wondered?

For a moment, I seemed caught in the pain and tragedy of those lives. Every one of these files had a name, a face, a family, and a sad story. Forgotten now, all but for the small paper trail they left behind.

Some even in death forgotten, forgotten by families who failed to claim their bodies when the end finally arrived. Forgotten and buried in the hospital cemetery beneath small grave markers that bore a number instead of a name.

And as if to add insult to injury, the cemetery that contains the bodies of over 1000 patients is presently missing, as lost and forgotten as the ones buried in its soil.

And then my thoughts turned to this: I could have been one of those files.

I sat down at a table next to Louise. This usually gregarious personality was quiet and withdrawn. I asked her again if she was okay, to which she responded with a nod.

Elaine brought in the files of Constance Margaret Fisher. They were contained in two folders, each about four inches thick. The volumes appeared to be worn, some even tattered.

I was now aware that others, perhaps many, had studied these documents to try to find out what made Constance Fisher tick, and explode.

The next three hours were a blur for me. It was my first window into a life of extreme complexity: one of joyful triumph and towering despair; an extremely private person who sought to be known and understood; a person who loved deeply, but was unable to love herself.

Many of the documents were stamped CONFIDENTIAL. I felt that I was viewing something very private, even sacred. I was entering the world of Constance Fisher as few had ever seen it, even family members.

Louise perused slowly, carefully through a small pile of documents from the early 1950's. She seemed to hang on every word.

How painful it must have been to re-live the nightmare of the tragedy and possibly make a discovery that could bring even more pain. I admired Louise for her courage and conviction to somehow bring purpose to her sisters pain, that perhaps Peggy's misfortune might lead to the absence of somebody else's.

We earmarked the documents we wanted, some 350 of them, which were copied and sent to Louise. She was then kind enough to send a copy to me for my research.

I was now able to make a detailed research of the files that contained patient interviews, evaluations, medical reports, observations, and letters home.

But it didn't take long to realize, however, that I was way over my head in trying to interpret test results and diagnostic labels. Fortunately, I had an expert opinion just a phone call away.

I phoned Dr. Jacobsohn that afternoon. He was joyful at my success in acquiring the records. I asked him if I could set up another appointment to talk, to which he agreed.

But first he asked if he could look at the documents and go over them before we talked. I was happy to oblige.

On September 28, I pulled into his residence with few answers and many questions. I brought lunch for Dr. Jacobsohn and his daughter Julie, herself a twenty-five year veteran in the mental health field. We barely got through the first course when the questions began and went rapid fire for the next two hours.

"There is one thing that troubles me about Mrs. Fisher," Dr. Jacobsohn said. "Her letters, in particular, reveal the absence of the ability to look outside of her illness, and look at it objectively. She never seemed at a place where she could look at her illness and say, 'I did something very bad and if I don't get help I could again do something awful.' Then, and then only, is a person no longer a risk to the community."

He said that the whole field of forensic psychiatry in the late 1950's was really still in its infancy, and that the staff at the Augusta State Hospital did not have much criteria in judging whether Constance was a viable candidate for release.

"The patient needs to be able to say ' I have to take responsibility for my own illness.' That should be the chief requirement for release. Connie Fisher never did that."

Dr. Jacobsohn recalled an incident in his practice when it did happen. It was with a patient who had been committed to AMHI for a violent outburst and treated successfully with Thorazine. After the situation was stabilized, however, his doctor and advocate recommended they discontinue the drug because of its side effects.

Despite the patient's protest, he was released without a prescription. He shortly fell into an episode in which he acquired a fire-arm, and in a rage shot the television set in his apartment, fired on the furniture, and then sent a volley through the window facing the street.

A stray bullet hit an elderly woman outside his apartment and killed her. The death was ruled accidental but he was tried with reckless homicide and re-committed to the Augusta Mental Health Institute.

He was held at the hospital for a number of years, exhibiting no signs of mental illness as long as he was on his medication. Based on his performance while taking medication, Dr. Jacobsohn was an advocate for the release of Henry Taylor.

As Dr. Jacobsohn stood before the bench awaiting the judge's decision on whether or not to allow Taylor back into the community, the judge pulled him aside and said, "We don't have another Constance Fisher here, do we?"

Dr. Jacobsohn said that the difference between the two was in how they dealt with their illness: one in denial, the other aware that he was sick and actively sought on-going treatment. Dr. Jacobsohn said the Henry Taylor case came to a happy conclusion. Taylor has continued to recover, and found his niche and place in society.

I told Dr. Jacobsohn that I could confirm his observation about Mrs. Fisher. The last recorded instance of any follow-up care from the Augusta State Hospital was September 12, 1960 when George Greeley visited the Fisher residence in Fairfield Center. Her file after that contained no record of any contact with the hospital save a birth notice that the Fishers sent to Dr. Sleeper on the birth of their daughter Kathleen in 1960.

No case worker, no follow up, and no request by Constance Fisher for evaluation or support. It spelled, and was, a recipe for disaster.

Curious, I asked Dr. Jacobsohn why he became a psychiatrist. He told the fascinating story of his upbringing as a Jew in Nazi Germany. He said that one day his father got a call from a medical school classmate at the University of Berlin, now a SS agent, who discovered the Jacobsohn name on a hit list, and that they were coming to get him and his family. In the space of an hour the family was on a train bound for Ethiopia.

"I had one relative who later worked on the Manhattan project and another who became a prominent member of the Luftwaffer," Dr. Jacobsohn said.

"How could that be if they were Jewish," I asked.

"Goering decided who was a Jew and who wasn't."

The family settled in Bangkok, Thailand, taking refuge in a Catholic monastery, where the elder Jacobsohn became an ophthalmologist. Persecuted for their race in Germany, the Jacobsohn's found themselves cultural outsiders in Thailand.

At the war's end, the family migrated to the United States where

Dr. Jacobsohn, without the benefit of a grade school or high school education, was accepted as a student at Reed College where he planned to follow his father's footsteps as an ophthalmologist. A hand tremor, however, caused him to make the painful decision to try another field of medicine. After working as an intern in a mental hospital, he decided to dedicate his life to the care of the mentally ill.

After successfully serving at mental hospitals and clinics in southern California, he went into private practice, while raising a family of four with his wife Jean. When they decided that southern California was not the best place to raise their family, Dr. Jacobsohn began looking for a new position.

In the summer of 1971, he met William Schumacher at a conference, who asked him to look into the possibility of filling a position at the Augusta State Hospital now known as the Augusta Mental Health Institute.

After doing some homework on the hospital, he became attracted to the rural setting and the hospital's historical significance. He then agreed to interview with Dr. James Patterson for a vacancy on the hospital staff.

Dr. Jacobsohn said he quickly fell in love with the facility, reminiscent to him of a college campus, with well-groomed landscapes, simple but friendly architecture, and a picturesque view of the Kennebec River. Before summers end, the family drove across country and took up residence in nearby Farmingdale.

Dr. Jacobsohn confessed that in the early 1970's, the Augusta Mental Health Institute was an institution in decline.

As I listened to his laundry list of problems, I harkened back to what Dr. Francis Sleeper had told newspaper men a generation before. It was essentially the same story; overcrowding, under-qualified and sometimes incompetent staff, and the frustration over the legislature being more interested in cutting costs than meeting needs.

He said that the institution was run on a shoe-string budget when reality called for an even greater financial commitment.

His first post at AMHI was overseeing the ranch ward, an area where patients did occupational therapy by learning farming techniques and maintaining the huge farm that had been a staple at the hospital since the beginning.

The farm had the residual benefit of producing produce, milk and eggs for the hospital and also the nearby veteran's hospital at Togus.

But then came a push by patients rights advocates, who said that the therapy was actually a type of slavery, and that the hospital was taking advantage of their labor by not paying them.

And although the therapeutic element of the program was never questioned, it was costly to maintain and the legislature was quick to dismantle it over the protest.

"It was a tragedy," Dr. Jacobsohn said of the death of the program. Patients were learning marketable skills and took great pride in the things they were learning and producing."

Dr. Jacobsohn's next post was overseeing the maximum security ward. It was first called the Criminally Insane Building and its construction grew out of a need to separate prisoners with mental illness from the rest of the patient population.

In 1907 the Maine legislature passed a measure to erect a facility on the campus that was down a considerable distance from the general population. The fortress-like structure had four stories, a floor for the least to the most violent.

Although they received treatment from the hospital staff, the prisoners living accommodations were bleak to say the least. This part of the hospital was perhaps most responsible for creating the negative image held by most of the public.

There was housing for about 40 patients, most of whom had committed capitol crimes or were deemed dangerous to the community.

The men lived dormitory style, in rows of the narrow cells with a place called " the cage" used for rebellious inmates. They enjoyed the light from one barred window, and were tucked in at night by the clank of an iron door and the twist of a key.

On the occasions when the men were allowed to go outside, it was on a small strip of land, about 200 by 100 feet, surrounded by an 18-foot wire fence tipped with razor wire. Even with that, 12 patients had escaped since 1953, the most recent Albert Paul, who was sent there for murder and was eventually found by state police hiding in the home of a hospital employee.

Their recreation and perhaps salvation, was in doing occupational therapy and repairing furniture used throughout the hospital.

It was there that Dr. Jacobsohn discovered Ernest M. Whittum, a lifer at the institution who had already been confined for 44 years. Whittum was accused, but never found guilty, of committing murder. Instead, at age 19, he had attempted to break into a home in Winterport, and was found guilty of breaking and entering and sentenced to three to six years of hard labor. In 1927, he was transferred to the Augusta State Hospital after he claimed he was hearing voices.

Unfortunately, his records did not accompany him, and a man who had only committed a petty crime was locked up in maximum security on the substance of a rumor that he had committed murder.

In 1971, reporter Elliot Jaspin for the Kennebec Journal, was sent to explore the Whittum case when hospital staff were unable to explain the few entries in his file or the nature of his crime. They could only prove that he had been transferred to the hospital in 1927, and that, unofficially there was talk that he had committed murder.

Jaspin then checked prison records at the Maine Corrections Center at Thomaston, leafed through 47-year-old editions of the Belfast Republican Journal and requested a review of the case by the Department of Mental Health and Corrections. When it came to the attention of Dr. Jacobsohn, who was now the acting superintendent of the hospital, immediate action was taken resulting in the transfer of Whittum to another part of the hospital and then his ultimate release.

Dr. Jacobsohn was quoted at the time as saying, that up to 50 percent of patients retained at the institution 20 years or longer would be better off in the community.

"I would do a review of patients like this every day," Jacobsohn said. "The Whittum case isn't that rare, only different in the way it came out."

The Whittum case gained national attention. He became known as the "Forgotten Man" and his case made institutions all over America evaluate their maximum security facilities that were often criticized as being " a place to hide society's undesirables" and providing little more than custodial care to those who were sentenced there.

Upon his release, Dr. Jacobsohn paid a visit to Whittum, who then was living in a rural northern Maine community.

"He was doing well," Dr. Jacobsohn told me. "Fishing, enjoying the company of his dog. He was not vindictive or seeking money or any other compensation by the state."

I asked Dr Jacobsohn why some fall through the cracks. "Some of it is the enormity and complexity of the case load and insufficient staff to handle it. It is a great responsibility one has in turning somebody free. You can be right 99% of the time and it is that one mistake that people will remember and hang you for."

Dr. Jacobsohn said that some of the blame also falls on the family or lack thereof. "Mrs. Fisher was fortunate in that respect; she always had visitors and a loving husband who was willing to take her back."

Before I left, Dr. Jacobsohn had some unexpected good news to relate. He had just returned from the annual meeting of the Academy of Psychiatry and the Law. Present at the meeting was Dr. Phillip Resnick, a noted expert in the field of forensic Psychiatry.

According to Dr. Jacobson he was the best, and had been called in to advise as an expert witness in such high profile cases as John Hinckley Jr., William Kennedy Smith, Jeffery Dahmer, Timothy McVeigh and pertinent to my interest, Andrea Yates.

Dr. Jacobsohn said that Dr. Resnick was familiar with the Fisher case, which I was beginning to understand was more than a just a series of rural Maine murders. It had national implications on how mentally ill criminals would be treated by the courts and by society.

Dr. Jacobsohn said he had spoken to Dr. Resnick about my research and secured a phone interview if I so desired it.

Φ Φ Φ Φ Φ Φ Φ Φ Φ Φ Φ Φ Φ Φ Φ Φ Φ Φ Φ

MY ACQUISITION OF CONSTANCE Fisher's medical records opened up new doors and gave the project instant credibility. I then decided to revisit some old sources, Dr. Loring Pratt in particular.

On August 7, I telephoned Dr. Pratt telling him that I had the documents and that I had already spoken with Dr. Jacobsohn. He said he would talk with me, but wanted to see at least a sample of the Fisher file. I was happy to oblige.

On August 12, I headed south up Interstate 95 to an appointment with Dr. Pratt on a beautiful sun drenched day. My thoughts turned to how such beauty could exists in such a fallen world, why there is such dichotomy between the perfection of the creation and the creatures who are called to be its chief steward. Fresh in my mind were images from a documentary on U.S. wars of the 20th century. Inventions such as tanks, artillery cannons, aerial bombs and finally the atomic bomb, had killed millions and left entire nations in ruin.

Brutal ground warfare left soldiers and civilians mentally and physically disfigured. The video presented methods of torture used to extract information that defied any definition of human decency.

The commentator speculated that of the millions who perished in the wars, there were even more to whom death would have come as a welcome relief.

Before I made it to Fairfield, I took the Waterville exit to visit the Miller Library at Colby College to check out a new lead.

I spoke briefly, and stated my business with the library clerk who seemed at first a little reluctant to help me. Was it my University of Maine windbreaker, or perhaps my graying hair that told her I was not exactly a student on campus?

When I mentioned that I was working on the Constance Fisher murder case however, she lit up.

"Oh yes, I know what you are talking about. Years ago, when I lived in Waterville, near the Catholic Cemetery, I used to walk my dogs towards the end of the cemetery. One day I looked up and saw an interesting headstone with three markers in the front and three markers in the back," she said before pausing to wait on a patron.

"It was that of a family, the Fisher family," she said. "The three headstones in the front were for three children, all with different birth dates but with the same death date. The same in the back, three markers for children, with different birth dates but the same death date. I always counted this very strange, until in the 1990's there was a woman in Texas who killed her children, Andrea Yates."

She mentioned that the Waterville Sentinel ran a piece on Mrs. Fisher telling of the murder of her two sets of children.

"And you are going to try to tell her story?," she asked.

"Yes, Ma'am, I am certainly going to try."

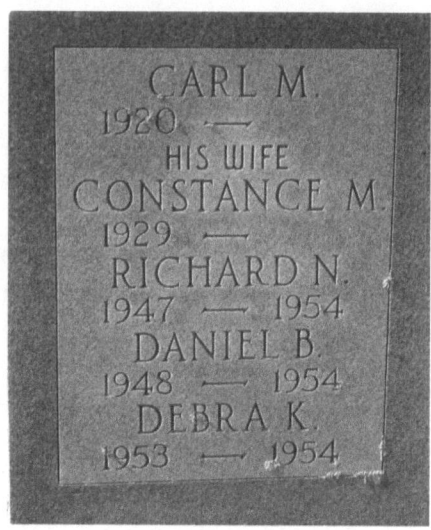

Fisher Memorial at the St. Francis Catholic Cemetery.

My time at the library also helped to get some information on former Waterville police chief, Albert Drost. Captain Drost had been the interrogating officer in both of the Fisher murder cases. Although I doubted he was still alive, I was hoping to find any information on him, perhaps an obituary, or where I could locate a next of kin.

I recovered enough information to get a sketch of a man who served his country and community well. He was of large physical stature with a commanding voice, surely an asset in most situations. He also possessed a compassionate and gentle side that allowed him to quiet defenses in others.

He served in various capacities for the Waterville Police Department from 1944-1969 and was a Kennebec County deputy sheriff. I also learned the name of his only child, Anna Bard, whom I interviewed over the phone.

Mrs. Bard said that she was living at her father's house when the first incident occurred in 1954, but she did not recall her father taking about it. She had married and was raising her own family when the second tragedy hit in 1966, but once again she remembered her father being mute on the topic.

"My father loved his career, but he was very closed-mouthed when it came to cases he worked on," she said. "He never brought things home, at least not that I can remember."

"But one this sensational, one of this notoriety," I questioned.

"I think my father had compassion for her. I think he realized that she did not know what she was doing, and if she was in her right mind would never have done it."

In perusing captain Drost's obituary, I noticed he was a World War II veteran and had fought in the battle of Okinawa.

The occupation of the small island of Okinawa was one of the bloodiest battles of the entire war. U.S. casualties alone would have outnumbered the entire population between Augusta and Bangor at the time.

It was known as the "Typhoon of steel" for the amount of bombs and ammunition used to capture the tiny but strategic parcel of ground.

It was combat at its fiercest and human kind at its most base element. Desperate hand-to-hand combat wounded and maimed, skies rained down bombs and bullets. Napalm bombs and flame throwers ousted families from their homes and soldiers from caves. Death marches were led for American prisoners who their captors did not want to feed, clothe, or care for. Beheading and dismemberment were common at the edge of Japanese Samaria.

Perhaps most criminal was the propaganda used by the Japanese soldiers to deceive the indigenous population whom they had previously used as human shields.

They told the natives that the American soldiers would rape, torture, and kill their children if they were victorious in battle.

Now I remembered it.

It was from the war documentary I had just finished viewing. It contained actual footage of an Okinawan mother throwing her children off a cliff to certain death on the rocks below after she learned of the American victory. Then she threw herself off.

She did so out of fear, thinking it in the best interest of her children as she believed the Americans were coming to torture them. It was not an act of murder, or insanity, but a deluded act of love and self-sacrifice based on nothing more than the lies of the Japanese soldiers.

Maybe what Constance Fisher did was not so horrific after all. She too had heard a lie spoken about the welfare of her children that she also believed and acted upon.

Φ Φ Φ Φ Φ Φ Φ Φ Φ Φ Φ Φ Φ Φ Φ Φ Φ Φ

I FOUND DR. PRATT SEATED in his study after being let in by his wife, Jeanette, who excused herself to go upstairs and finish the ironing.

Through the archives in my own mind I had pieced some history together that I had with Dr. Pratt many years ago.

He was one of the leading ear, nose, and throat specialists in central Maine when I was a boy, a fact that did not escape my mother who was a registered nurse. I had severe allergy problems as a child and had been to see Dr. Pratt who removed my tonsils to solve the symptoms.

Since they are no longer considered a vestigial organ, I politely asked Dr. Pratt if I could have my tonsils back, to which he responded, " Yes, if you can find them."

Dr. Pratt invited me to pull up a chair and I showed him a collection of the documents I had received from Louise Bowker and the signed release form. It seemed to satisfy him, that he was now free to tell me all he knew about Mrs. Fisher.

"I did not know her socially," Dr. Pratt began. "Even though they were part of this community, I never saw her except for the one time."

My heart dropped. I was running out of source people that actually knew the Fishers, especially in their own town. I was curious to understand the feeling around town, what people thought of her, how they treated her… and did they forgive her?

"I am sorry, but I cannot answer any of those questions for you," Dr. Pratt continued.

I began to wonder if anyone could. After obtaining the medical records, I had all the information on her physical and mental condition I could have hoped for. It was the anecdotal information that I was hoping Dr. Pratt might supply.

"But I did see her once professionally," Dr. Pratt interjected.

He said that sometime during the first week of March, 1954, Carl and Constance Fisher came to his office in the professional building on 177 Main Street in Waterville. Their children did not accompany them.

He described Constance as a trim, attractive woman, soft spoken and polite. He described Mr. Fisher as, tall, thin "a pleasant, soft-spoken gentleman."

Coming at the recommendation of Dr. Richard Chasse, Mrs. Fisher complained to him of an inner ear problem which Dr. Pratt diagnosed as an infection in the ear canal.

He cleaned out her ear with a wick and a local antiseptic and gave her an antibiotic to take home. He then explained that conditions such as this can be caused by scalp problems such as eczema or dandruff and that he would write her a prescription for a special shampoo.

He cautioned her to use the shampoo judiciously, however. He said it contained a poisonous element that could be fatal if swallowed.

He warned Constance not to touch any food after handling the shampoo, clean up thoroughly after using it, even cleaning under her fingernails. He warned most importantly to keep it away from the children.

"And then, as they were leaving, Carl Fisher said that they had to hurry to catch another appointment, with a Dr. Jones in Union," Dr. Pratt said. "I knew Dr. Jones, that he was a psychiatrist. This was my first indication that something might have been wrong with her."

Dr. Pratt said that as soon as they left his office, he placed a phone call to Dr. Jones, warning him that he may have written Mrs. Fisher an instrument of destruction.

On Tuesday, February 9, 1954, the sad news landed on Dr. Pratt's door step that Mrs. Fisher had drowned her three children and had tried to kill herself by drinking the bottle of Selsum shampoo that he had prescribed.

In a hospital interview, dated March 25, 1954, Mrs. Fisher explained her actions:

> "…. I found a bottle of poison and that was what I took but it did not work. It was a very poisonous shampoo. It was on the label that it was so poisonous that after you use it you should clean your hands carefully even brush to get it from under the nails, but it must be exaggerated because it did not work…."

The news was as shocking to Dr. Pratt as it was to the rest of the community.

"Needless to say, I was upset," he continued. I was sad for her. There was nothing at the appointment in her talk or manner that would have pointed to anything like this. She was quiet and polite, but in retrospect I could see that she may have been depressed."

I asked again if there was anything about her that might have suggested she was struggling with emotional problems.

"She seemed a little depressed and as I mentioned she was on her way to see Dr. Jones. But there was certainly nothing to indicate that she was a menace to herself or anyone else."

I asked him, given the way the situation played out, if those who treated her mental illness should have done anything different.

"I am not a psychiatrist" Dr. Pratt answered. This is a question outside of my expertise."

* CHAPTER EIGHT *

WHY?

"In that day we will know fully as we were fully known.

Paul to the Corinthians, 57 AD

Iₙ July of 2009, a filicide hit a town in New Jersey where a 38-year-old mother shot her 4-month old son, then attempted to kill her boyfriend before turning the gun on herself. The diagnosis and reason given for the tragedy: Post Partum Depression.

In the newspaper article describing the tragedy, friends and relatives were mystified by the young mother's actions. She didn't have a police record, she didn't drink, do drugs, was reported to be a good mother and a good employee.

Once again, the evidence that defined the person did not add up to the crime.

Many of the readers commenting on the crime had already raced to judgment, taking the act at face value only. Many felt the crime so heinous that even ending her own life was not punishment enough.

One blogger wrote:

"A sin. I am so ticked off right now I can not even respond…
I am trying to get myself together because I do not wish people to

Hell but you killed your 4 month old child? Why didn't you just kill yourself if you wanted to die..."

Others wrote:

"Witch...Crazy....Burn in Hell...senseless act of murder. There is no excuse for what she did. The bottom line is that she killed a four month old baby."

"She was probably drunk and mad at the world for some reason and once she realized what she had done, she probably thought suicide would be preferable to spending life in prison..."

"Listen to all these people make excuses for this violent woman that shoots her boy friend and then shoots and kills her son... Women are the most violent persons out there and until law enforcement realizes that women are the cause of most domestics they will never resolve the problem. Poor kid."

But another wrote:

"One can only imagine the torment and the pain a mother must have been experiencing to take her child's life and then her own. We must find mercy in our hearts... If the harsh judgments expressed in this forum are any indication of the world at large it is not difficult to see why this poor woman took it to the brink."

I wondered if people a generation ago felt the same way about the Fisher murders.

America was at a different place then to be sure. From the little I could garner, Mainers seemed much more compassionate and were willing to give Mrs. Fisher another chance, at least after the first tragedy.

I was also interested to know what people present day thought of the Fisher murders.

I conducted a survey soliciting information from as diverse a pool as I could get. I interviewed people in several states and from a cross section of ages, occupations, and value systems. (1)

The survey read as follows:

****

Your occupation: _____

Question:

After Mrs. Fisher killed her children in 1954, she should have been:

A. Given capitol punishment.
B. Sentenced to life in prison.
C. Committed to a mental hospital
D. If cured, returned to the community.

Comments:

****

The results of the survey are as follows:

> **Capitol Punishment - 60%**
> **Committed to a Mental Hospital - 23%**
> **Life in Prison - 15%**
> **Returned to Community if cured - 2%**

When told that upon release Mrs. Fisher murdered again:

> **Capitol Punishment - 90%**
> **Life in Prison - 8%**
> **Committed to a Mental Hospital - 2%**
> **Returned to Society if cured - 0%**

More insightful than the numbers were the comments:

> **Police officer**
> Capitol punishment
> *"If they kill their own children they are never going to be cured in their mind."*

Athletic trainer
Commitment to a mental hospital
*"There is nothing my children could ever do
that would make me even think of killing them. There is no way
you could do that and not be mentally ill."*

Teacher
Life in prison
*"For her to get off scott-free sets a poor precedent for society which
is much too lenient. Because of the nature of the crime, you need
to be positively sure it will never happen again and you can't be.
And what about the kids…who is going to give them a second
chance?"*

Basketball official
Capitol punishment
*"She should have been sent to Iraq or Afghanistan (Korea or
Vietnam in this case) to repay her debt to society. If cured she
should have been re-tried… I'll tell you what the problem is, too
many rights."*

Health care professional
Capitol punishment
*"Multiple murderers should be given death. People are always
blaming the drug or the sickness or the devil for killing and worse.
There is an element of human responsibility involved in murder.
Hypnotism has proved that you cannot do a deed unless it is given
permission in your psyche."*

Elementary school teacher
Committed to a mental hospital
*"What is the difference between what Mrs. Fisher did and a
mother killing her child by a saline abortion? The only difference
is that the child suffers for a much longer period during one of
those."*

Superior Court Judge
Committed to a mental hospital
"Unfortunately, I deal with these situations every week. It must

be understood that under our law one is innocent until proven guilty. Often, the first response is to pronounce guilty until proven innocent."

Stem cell biologist
Returned to society.
"If you can say that she is definitely cured than she should have a second chance and return to society."

Radiologist
Mental Hospital or prison
"God, it's kids... There is no way she should get out. And how can you determine or declare someone to be cured? For the second time around, capitol punishment... The people in charge, the ones who made the decisions own their share of guilt and should have been held responsible.

Law student
Committed to a mental hospital
"The concept of pardon is not foreign to our society or judicial system. Measures could have been taken however, such as sterilization, that the incident not be repeated. My question is, was there an ulterior motive in letting her go?"

Middle School counselor
Committed to a mental hospital
"If she did it once she is capable of doing it again. Anyone who drowns their own or any child has had a real break from reality. She should never get out and even have the possibility of doing it again. It was children, we do not do enough to protect our children."

Maine guide
Returned to society
"If that's the way the system works than so be it. It is not infallible, mistakes are made. Prisoners are paroled all the time and then commit crimes. What makes this crime seem so heinous is that it involves children."

Accountant
"Can I give you a fifth option? If cured, go to jail for life. Personal responsibility at some point has got to come into play. We hear too much of the time 'I am not responsible because of my...' The reason why is not important. If you did the crime you should pay the price."

Contractor
Committed to a mental hospital
"She should be put away so it could never happen again. She should be given the help she needs but still incarcerated. And how do you know if she is cured. There is the possibility it could happen again. Past history is a good indicator of future behavior."

Police detective
Capitol punishment
"This is a classic case of an outcome that should have been determined by the judicial system instead of psychiatrists that know nothing about criminal law and criminal behavior."

Musician
Committed to a mental hospital
"Self love, not love for the children. It sounds like she was an insecure mother and insecure in her marriage. Her act was the ultimate betrayal in every way, shape and form. The husband is almost equal in his guilt; there were warning signs all over the map. She bought the end result by listening to Satan."

Researcher
Life in prison
"First, capitol punishment should never be an option even for capitol crimes. And even though we forgive her, there still needs to be a punishment but a punishment that best suits the crime.

Insurance agent
Capitol punishment
"Why should we be burdened with maybe paying $45,000 a year for her crimes against humanity...?"

Grade school student
Capitol punishment
"The punishment should fit the crime, an eye for an eye, tooth for a tooth. There is no excuse for a crime that bad. The crime needs to be punished, and if she was let out how could her husband ever trust her to be alone with the kids?"

Barber
Capitol punishment
"I was cutting hair in Waterville when the murders happened in the 1960's. Another barber I was talking to had the solution. He said she should have drowned herself with the first batch of children. I always wondered what kind of a hold she had over her husband."

Engineer
Committed to a mental hospital
"You have to do what is right for the society. The rights of the many have to trump the rights of the few. The liberty of one individual ends where the end of another's nose begins. This dynamic creates some of the greatest ethical dilemmas a society must face."

High school Sunday school student
Committed to a mental hospital
"I guess, what would Jesus do? I think He would reach out in compassion and mercy but would say 'go and sin no more.' Also, God sees differently than we do. He knows all the facts, all the factors, discerns and sees everything. And there is probably a whole lot that people don't know about this case."

Writer
Committed to a mental hospital
"It seems to me that too many of the people at the top, the ones controlling the decision making process, need more education in the real world. They have more degrees than a thermometer but get a failing grade in common sense. The trauma Mrs. Fisher must have felt every time she saw a bathtub, every time she saw an infant or young children, every time she saw the grief in the eyes of her husband, should have been punishment enough."

Mental health nurse
Committed to a mental hospital
"She has already suffered enough. When a patient returns to normalcy, especially after committing a crime like this, it is something they can never forget. They are in prison, a prison in their own mind. The people who judge and condemn have no idea how tortured these individuals really are."

Assistant attorney general
Committed to mental hospital
"Imagine what it must take for a person, especially a mother, to do that. It tempers your outrage when you think about what frame of mind she must have been in. I interviewed her (Mrs. Fisher) and I recall having a great deal of compassion for her… I can't imagine how anyone, after killing three children, ever having the opportunity to kill three more."

Health care professional
Committed to a mental hospital
"There is such a connection between the mind and the body. I used to think that it would be impossible to do any harm to anybody, no less your own children, but now I am not so sure. Given the right circumstances anyone is capable of doing almost anything."

Pastor
Returned to society
"She should be released if proved to be cured. However, if she had a spiritual problem, a spirit can't be talked out, shocked out, or be medicated out. They have to be driven out."

Probably my most insightful interview came from an Augusta doctor in private practice.

He agreed that in some cases, capitol punishment is an appropriate answer, but not in this one. Because she had a certifiable mental illness, that should have excluded her.

When asked if the mental health system had failed Mrs. Fisher he said no, "Mrs. Fisher failed Mrs. Fisher."

He questioned the call of the mental health professionals who were willing to give her a second chance.

"Good old-fashioned common sense would tell you that you don't give a person who committed so heinous a crime the opportunity to do it again, you don't set the table for her again. In my experience, having dealt, on occasion, with similar situations, she was too dangerous a threat to be released back into the community, no less allowed to have more children. We have laws on the books and it is a priority of the government to protect the people. There are certain types of criminal behavior that should never be released.

What she did was beyond crazy, against every instinct in her being to kill her own children. You don't need 11 years of higher education to figure that one out. To even give her the opportunity to do it again was a breach in judgment, especially where illnesses of the mind are so unpredictable.

This was, in many ways, a landmark case because it changed the insanity defense, and also the concept of having proper follow-up, especially in high-profile cases when that one error in judgment can cast a shadow on the whole profession."

His diagnosis was that Mrs. Fisher was a sociopath which might account for why she seemingly had little or no remorse over the killings, only when it was to her advantage.

"A sociopath is one of society's greatest manipulators and can convince anybody of anything. She obviously did that to the medical panel and probably her own husband and family.

The stigma that surrounds mental illness is tragic and prohibits treatment for many who need it. If you are physically ill, you are treated with sympathy. If you are mentally ill, you are treated with scorn.

I have a great concern for those who are not being treated, and have been cut loose by the hospitals and are out on the streets. There are untreated people out there, maybe many, who are capable of doing just about anything at any time."

Φ Φ Φ Φ Φ Φ Φ Φ Φ Φ Φ Φ Φ Φ Φ Φ Φ Φ

A PARENT KILLING THEIR OFFSPRING? While head scratching, it has a history as old as mankind itself. Infanticide, a catch-all term for all types of child homicide, has been practiced world wide and by every culture. It was practiced by the Pharaoh of Egypt to exterminate the Jewish race. It was practiced by the Romans to get rid of the Christ child. It is practiced in China for population control. It is practiced in America to terminate unwanted pregnancy.

It has been practiced by peoples at every level of civilization, sometimes being the rule and not the exception.

Under Roman law, a father exercised absolute rule over his household. The murder of illegitimates, females, or excess children was rarely questioned by authorities. It was merely part of the "patria potens," the rights of the head of the household.

A letter home from a Roman soldier in the first century records this sentiment:

> *"I am still in Alexandria. I beg and plead with you to take care of our little child, and as soon as we receive wages I will send them to you. In the meantime (if fortune is good to you) and you give birth, if it's a boy, let it live; if it's a girl, expose it."*

Dr. Philip J. Resnick, author and professor of Psychiatry and Director of Forensic Psychiatry at Case Western Reserve University School of Medicine, has spent years studying the problem of filicide, and is considered a leading expert in the field. (2)

Dr. Resnick says that filicides occur in approximately 3% of all homicides in the United States. He said the most dangerous period for the victim is within the first year of life, a time when post-partum psychosis and depression are often experienced.

And significantly, 50 % or more of women who had a previous episode of post-partum depression experience a relapse after a subsequent pregnancy. The relapse rate for post partum psychosis is close to 80%.

Resnick writes that mothers with post-partum depression are often reluctant to share their emotions or feeling towards the child for fear that others might think of them as a bad mother. Society views women as innate nurturers who are expected to remain happy throughout their pregnancy and motherhood.

He said that methods of filicide differ and are different according to sex. Mothers who kill their offspring usually choose suffocation, strangulation, and drowning. Fathers tend to use more forceful means such as blows to the head, bludgeoning, or stabbing.

Perhaps one of the best-known filicides committed by a father in the 20th century, was at the hand of a professional baseball player named Martin Bergen.

On Friday morning, January 10, 1900, Bergen viciously killed his wife and children, bludgeoning them to death with an axe before nearly decapitating himself with a straight razor.

Aged 28, and about to reach his prime as a ball player, Bergen was known as a gentle, attentive, husband and loving father of two. He had reached out in vain for the help of physicians prior to the act.

His obituary in a Boston paper read:

North Brookfield, Mass, Jan 10

> *Martin Bergen one of the best known ball players in the country and one of the Boston clubs catchers last season, killed his wife and two children with an axe and then cut his own throat with a razor. When the father of the murderer and suicide entered the house today, Martin Bergen's body and those of the little girl, Florence, six and one half years old, were laying on the kitchen floor while in the adjoining bedroom were the bodies of Mrs. Bergen and her three year old son, Joseph. Mrs. Bergen was lying on the bed with her hands raised as if in supplication or trying to ward off a blow. The little boy was lying on the floor with a large wound in the head. Mrs. Bergen's skull was terribly crushed having evidently been struck more than one blow by the infuriated husband. The appearance of the little girl also showed that a number of savage blows had been rained upon the top and side of her head. Bergen's throat had been cut with a razor and the head was nearly severed from the body.*

Bergen's brother Bill, also a major league ball player, was quoted as saying, "It was as if he was possessed. The ghosts got to him and never let him go."

Dr. Resnick classifies filicides according to motive, citing six reasons why a mother or a father would kill their own child:

-**Spousal revenge**, where a husband or a wife will destroy that which is most precious to their spouse.

-**Fatal maltreatment**, where neglect or abuse claims the life of the child.

-**Acutely psychotic**, where the act is a product of mental illness and the perpetrator feels compelled to act by a force outside themselves.

-**Altruistic**, where the goal is to relieve the suffering, real or imagined, of a child or children. It is usually accompanied by suicide or a suicide attempt.

Dr. Resnick also notes that severe depression, even without psychotic features, may so distort thinking that a mother believes her children will be much better off in the next life.

In addressing command hallucinations, Resnick said that the voice is more likely to be obeyed if the voice is familiar.

Responding to a command hallucination thought to be God, is perceived as being the right thing to do. In addition, the parent may feel unable to refrain because the command is from God.

Dr. Resnick was called as an expert witness in the case of Andrea Yates, who killed her five children believing that God had commanded her to do it. Although initially found guilty and sentenced to life in prison, a later appeal found her innocent by reason of insanity and she was committed to the care of a mental health facility.

Dr. Resnick noted several similarities between the Constance Fisher and Andrea Yates cases:

- Drowning was the mode of death.
- The eldest child was found face down in the tub, while the others were wrapped in blankets or sheets and laid on their beds.
- Both left notes that expressed their love for the children with the hope that they were in a better place.
- Both acted contrary to their moral code.
- Both believed that God had commanded them to kill their children.

One of the few who could have genuine empathy for the Yates tragedy was Louise Bowker.

She wrote a letter to Russell Yates, the father of the five dead children that was never answered.

"I've been trying all week to think of how to tell him that we know the pain he is going through," she told a newspaper reporter shortly after the tragedy.

* CHAPTER NINE *

DR. ISAAC RAY

"But if insanity depends upon disease of the brain, as is now universally admitted, the question may be pertinently asked, why should it not be equally under the control of medicines, and treated upon with the same general principals as other bodily diseases?"

Dr. Isaac Ray, 1842

THAT CONSTANCE FISHER WAS not convicted of murder and sentenced to prison for the rest of her life, she had former Maine Insane Hospital superintendent Dr. Isaac Ray to thank.

At a time when the treatment of those suffering with mental illness was emerging from the dark, it was Dr. Ray who gave them a medical standing before the demands of justice.

Dr. Ray is called the father of American forensic psychiatry. He was one of the original 13 founding members of the Association of Medical Superintendents of American Institutions for the Insane (later the American Psychiatric Association), where he served as president for many years.

He was one of the most quoted authors in his field in the 19th and 20th centuries, publishing over one hundred works.

Dr. Ray was one of the first expert witnesses to appear in the courtroom to help decide in cases that involved mental illness.

And it was Dr. Ray who gave modern society it's first working definition of mental illness as it pertained to forensic psychiatry:

"A departure from the ordinary character and habits of a person without any adequate motive or stimulus." (1)

He was among the first modern psychiatrists to recognize the difference between the brain and the mind. He defined the brain as an organ, and the mind as its manifestation.

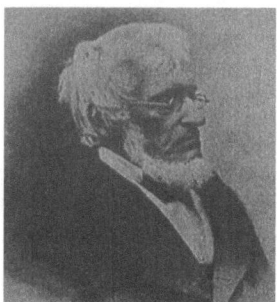

Dr. Isaac Ray c. 1875.
Dr. Ray was the second superintendent at the Maine Insane Hospital. He has been internationally acclaimed for his work in forensic psychiatry.

Born in Massachusetts in 1807, Ray moved to Maine after graduating from Phillips Academy in 1822. He went on to attend Bowdoin College and Bowdoin College School of Medicine and Surgery. There he rubbed shoulders with some of the country's greatest intellectuals of the period: authors Nathaniel Hawthorne and Henry Wadsworth Longfellow, historian Jacob Abbott, and future U.S. president Franklin Pierce. Ironically, Pierce would later oppose Ray's efforts to establish mental hospitals on a land grant basis.

After graduating from Bowdoin, Ray set up practice in Portland, Maine in 1827. Unable to build a general practice there, he moved to Eastport where he took on work as a public lecturer, book reviewer, and author.

In Eastport, Ray began to focus his study on the diseases of the mind. He took a particular interest in the writings of Sir Francis Bacon and the French physician, Philippe Pineal, who both viewed mental illness as simply being a disease of the bodily organ called the brain.

Slowly, his concept of the brain and mental illness began to crystallize. Revolutionary at the time, Ray began to speak and write that diseases of the brain were like that of any other organ. And like any other organ, the brain works dependently and in synergy with other parts.

This allowed Ray to dispel the notion that mental disease was a meta-physical problem, a character defect, or a moral failing. It was a disease that attacks and ravages the brain like consumption would the lungs.

Ray believed that the only obstacle to curing mental illness was a lack of knowledge of the brains operation and the curative agents to which it would respond.

Ray concluded that the mind then depended upon the entire body for its manifestation and advocated that the study of the body, primarily through autopsy, might provide some clues as to why it malfunctions.

Ray lobbied Maine legislators for the use of cadavers in experimentation, citing laws in Massachusetts that enabled the corpses of criminals and paupers for dissection.

He was quoted in the May 31, 1831 Portland Daily Courier as saying:

> *People expect great knowing and skill from their doctor but they withhold the very means of acquiring either. Society expects the doctor to have the most minute acquaintance with the intricate and beautiful mechanism of the human structure, yet if he attempts to examine one of these wonderful machines he is prosecuted as a criminal and driven from society.*

Ray also labored to debunk the myth that the mentally ill were somehow predestined to lives of torture by Divine Providence. Like Bacon, he believed that it was God's will that the secrets of the universe be discovered through careful and unprejudiced observation for the betterment of all mankind.

Ray believed that mental illness could have both a physical and environmental trigger, which he called causes.

He labeled the first a "constitutional cause," or one caused by heredity, or a " predisposition to the disease founded on some organic peculiarity not well understood."

The second he labeled an environmental, or "exciting cause," an event, behavior, or circumstance that caused the upset.

He later catalogued a list of exciting causes:

Use of tobacco, opium
Sexual deviance
Lack of physical and mental exercise
Too much study
Lack of relaxation
Lack of sleep
Lack of a proper diet
Stress, emotional and environmental
Disease in other body organs
Lack of fresh air
Negative outlook on life
Worries about the future

Dr. Ray also became a student of phrenology, a theory that espoused that personality and other traits could be measured by examining the size and shape of a person's skull.

Phrenology to Ray provided the bridge between spiritually based theories of the mind and the material concept that he was now embracing. It had a large following across America in the 19th century, with proponents ranging from quack physicians who would read "bumps" at county fairs, to serious medical scholars like Ray.

The phrenologist held that areas in the brain have specific, localized functions. Thus, it could be said that the brain was made up of many separate organelles that comprised the one organ.

It was believed that the cranial bone conformed in order to accommodate the different sizes of these areas of the brain so that a person's capacity for a given personality trait could be determined simply by measuring the area of the skull that overlies the corresponding region.

The phrenologist would run his hands over a patient for bumps and indentations in order to get a reading. By making reference to a phrenology map, he could then determine if a potential mate, employee, or business partner would be of suitable disposition.

A good phrenology map identified the location of 27 "brain organs" that controlled activities such as, religiosity, memory, language, love of ones offspring, and the tendency to murder.

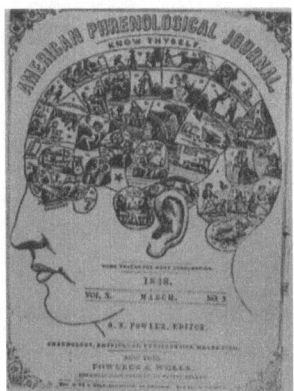

**Phrenology helped Dr. Ray to estimate the inner workings of the brain.
Thomas Edison said it helped him to discover his inventive abilities.
Sir Arthur Conan Doyle advocated it in several of his writings.
Phrenology charts were later supplemented by the Automatic
Electric Phrenometer to make more precise readings.**

Phrenology also helped Ray to understand how a patient could be positively rational in many areas of thought but deviant in others, sometimes only one.

What Ray was learning in theory, however, he lacked in experience. Only occasionally in his general practice would he encounter a psychiatric patient, but that would change dramatically in 1841.

After only six months at the Maine Insane Hospital, Cyrus Knapp, the institutions first superintendent, suddenly left the hospital. Officials looked no further than their own state to find a replacement.

Dr. Ray's book, "Treatise on the Medical Jurisprudence of Insanity," was gaining him national acclaim, and he became the popular choice to replace Knapp.

Dr. Ray had little idea of what awaited him at the new, state of the art facility, as he traveled by stage across state from Eastport to Augusta.

He was about to learn of the magnitude of the problem of mental illness in Maine and how deep into the abyss of human suffering that some of its victims had fallen.

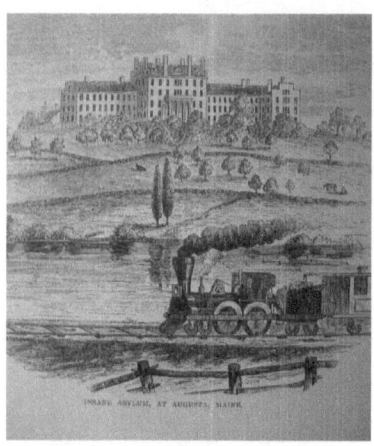

**Newspaper sketch of the Maine Insane Hospital, about 1850.
Courtesy Maine Historic Preservation.**

Upon his arrival, Dr. Ray found everything at the hospital turn-key and ready to go. Ready to go with one notable exception; he had very few patients. But Dr. Ray knew that the state had many more individuals in need of the hospital's care. He wrote in the 1841 year end superintendents report that:

> *The first point that arrests our attention is the comparably small number of the insane that have been received into the Hospital. By the Untied States census of 1840 it appears that there are in this state 631 insane persons of which number only 135 have enjoyed at all the benefits of the institution. Of these 631 person, a large portion, no doubt are idiots and other incurables, who can hardly be considered as fit subjects of medical or moral treatment and who are as well off wherever they are kindly treated, as they would be with us...*
>
> *Still, after making all reasonable deductions of this kind, there are unquestionably more than 135 who would be either completely restored or greatly improved mentally and bodily by a residence in the Hospital.*

Rays first order of business was to sell the idea of the hospital to the public and to the Maine legislature.

It would be a tough sell. Mental illness was a problem that most Mainers would rather not talk about, or even admit existed. It was the inconvenient truth of that era.

The legislature skeptically viewed the hospital as an experiment, and one most likely to fail. They figured that if the enterprise went under, the land could always be sold and the building converted into another utility.

Ray abhorred the terms "lunatic asylum" or "nut house" that some used to describe the hospital.

He labored to promote the facility as a hospital, not a dumping grounds, or place of incarceration and exile. Here the sick would come to be treated, held as long as it took to be cured, then returned promptly to their communities and homes.

A pioneer in an emerging field, Ray had no predecessor and little history to draw from in running the hospital.

He began networking with superintendents of other pioneering hospitals, sharing information on diagnosis, treatments, and the nuts and bolts of running the new enterprise.

By 1843, Ray had settled in at the hospital and patients were coming from all quarters of the state, being brought to Augusta by sailing ships, stage coaches, and horseback. From his residence in the Stone Building he could keep tabs on the entire hospital where it is said he knew every patient and every worker by name.

Looking out the south windows of his third story flat, Dr, Ray could see the hospital farm and the acres of tilled soil yielding vegetables and fruits to service the needs of the hospital. He viewed the selling of surplus crop as a financial safety net should the legislature choose at any point to cut back funding.

Ray believed there was a great benefit for patients to be out in the fresh air and sunshine, gaining a sense of accomplishment as they worked toward recovery. He wrote:

> We consider the farm connected with the Hospital of very great importance to the interests and success of the institution. Employment of some kind is essential to the recovery of the insane and even to the keeping of a well person sane. Confinement without employment is enough to drive any and all to madness.
>
> No employment is so congenial to the human constitution as agriculture. Man was made "to till the ground." Agriculture furnishes the most healthful exercise and enables the operator to breathe the pure air of heaven.

It is not designed that labor should be compulsive, but entirely voluntary on the part of patients.

Looking east, from the back windows of his dwelling, Dr. Ray could observe the area that was turning into ball fields for the new sport known as baseball invented by Abner Doubleday a few years earlier in Cooperstown, New York. He rightly discerned the value of organized recreation as a way to channel harmful inward energies to an outward expression that had the fringe benefit of being fun.

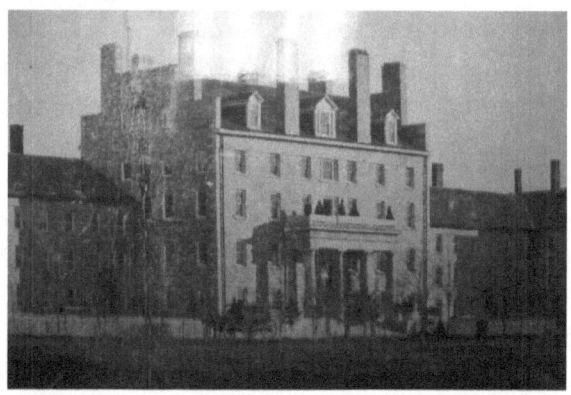

Spectators enjoy the view off the superintendents portico at the Maine Insane Hospital, c. 1860. Courtesy Maine Historic Preservation.

From the windows facing west, Dr. Ray had a view of the Kennebec River, the supreme artery for commerce for central Maine, with business and recreational boating in the summer, and ice harvesting and ice fishing in the winter. In the background stood the village of Augusta that had, a little over a decade ago, become the capitol city of Maine.

To the north, Dr. Ray could view flower gardens and other ornamental horticulture, their sight and fragrances also believed to be therapeutic. He could see the stable for the horse and carriage used to take patients on Sunday drives around the countryside and river bank.

Ray himself was enhanced intellectually by the appealing surroundings. From his living and work space, he wrote a second and expanded edition of his book, "Treatise on the Medical Jurisprudence of Insanity."

Ray would add other tenets of moral treatment during his tenure at the hospital. He established a library, enlarged space for a chapel, and had music performed and taught.

Dr. Ray was open to any concept that might exact a positive change in his patients. All of the healing arts, including prayer, were welcomed at the hospital. He wrote that:

> *Proper diet, exercise, change of air and scene, lead to a useful and agreeable occupation of the mind… In many cases some amusement or other is the first thing that arrests the attention and withdraws the mind for a moment from the contemplation of its own morbid fanaticizes…*
>
> *Combining physical with mental exercise it has been found more productive than any other for cheerfulness, good spirits and diversion of the thoughts into healthier channels.*

During his four-year stint, Dr. Ray developed more than a hospital. The Maine Insane Hospital became a therapeutic community, modeled after the human body itself.

It was a place which had various moving parts, each performing its own function, but working in synergy toward the end of making patients whole again, body, mind, and spirit.

Dr. Ray's second crusade was to change the injustice done to the mentally ill cast into jails and prisons. He pitied the plight of those incarcerated for offenses that were the result of illness, not a breach of morality.

Behind bars, they often received the antithesis of moral treatment. They were beaten, whipped into submission, and kept in damp cells and cages.

It was for such that Ray scoured the local prisons, looking for those condemned for acts committed while under the influence of their disease.

It was during one of these trips that he found Moses Butterfield, jailed at the county prison in Paris, after committing one of the first recorded filicides in the state.

Butterfield, a citizen of repute in his hometown of Sumner, had killed his wife and three of his children with an axe in a psychotic rage in 1841.

The April, 1841 edition of the Kennebec Journal gave the following account of the tragedy:

Paris, Oxford County, April 25

There has been a sad tragedy acted this week in the next town of which I will give you the particulars. Mr. Moses Butterfield of Sumner, has been for a number of years subject to fits of partial derangement, not so as to render him incapable of attend to his affairs, but he runs of strange notions.

Last Wednesday he killed his wife and two children one aged two and the other nine years, and wounded a third so that her recovery is considered doubtful. He came into his house with an axe and commenced his work of slaughter by striking his wife as she sat knitting on the back of her neck. As she fell from her chair she called to a daughter to help her up- the daughter ran to assist her dying mother and met the maniac with the uplifted axe.

She fled out of the house and ran to the nearest neighbors Capt. Jesse Howes. When Mr. H arrived at Butterfield's he found him sitting on a chest with a number of sharpened knives by him. When asked why he had done so he said it was his duty to kill his family, and that he was going to cut his own throat if Mr. H. had not come in.

The child that is living which he wounded ran to the barn and up a ladder. He followed her knocked her off, struck her on the neck with the axe and left her; when found she had crawled under the straw. She is 11 years old.

One little son six years old ran for the woods where two older brothers where at work making sugar. His father followed him but stopping to pick up his hat which had fallen off, the child was enabled to run to the woods and escaped by concealing himself behind a stump.

The wretched man is in jail and still declares he must kill the rest of his family, though he talks rational about other matters. He had eight children.

We have confirmation of the above by a person from Sumner in this town with details too horrid for description. The wretch chopped off the heads of his wife and children with an axe and when the alarm was given by his child which had escaped, and assistance arrived, he was holding the bloody head of his child in his hand and made no effort to escape.

Although Butterfield was acquitted by reason of mental defect, he was sentenced to a fate perhaps worse than death; life in prison with no hope of parole or treatment. There, he could expect to be tormented for his crime by prison officials and inmates alike.

Butterfield languished in the jail for three years before he was rescued by Dr. Ray and transported by stage across state to the Maine Insane Hospital.

An 1846 report listed Butterfield as the 350th patient at the hospital, having been there since May 26, 1844. His condition was listed as improved but his diagnosis read incurable.

Despite the diagnosis, the sentence, and at one time testifying of a mission to kill the remainder of his family, Moses Butterfield was released from the hospital after doctors considered him cured.

Unfortunately, he had a flare-up of his disease, but voluntarily committed himself to the Maine Insane Hospital where he spent the rest of his life, dying, in 1865, at age 76.

This incident, and another that followed, brought to light the vexing problem of when, or if, a forensic patient should be released.

Dr. Ray held two things to be most important in the treatment process: that patients be brought to the hospital at the very onset of symptoms, and secondly, they remain there until the process of recovery was completed.

In 1841, towns had voted to send patients to the institution for a specified length of time, when patients would be removed regardless of their condition. Ray argued that patients who had been troubled for years would sometimes take years to get well. Premature release would only increase their chance of relapse and a return to the institution, or worse.

This issue would surface in 1850, when a patient that had been admitted to the hospital during Ray's tenure and prematurely released, wrote a sensational essay that received national attention.

Titled, **"Three Years in a Mad House by a Victim,"** Isaac H. Hunt sought to victimize Dr. Ray and the institution for its "barbaric behaviors and treatments."

The publications cover bore the image of Hunt being held to the floor by three attendants while Ray stood over him. The caption read, ***"Dr. Ray giving Poisonous Medicines."***

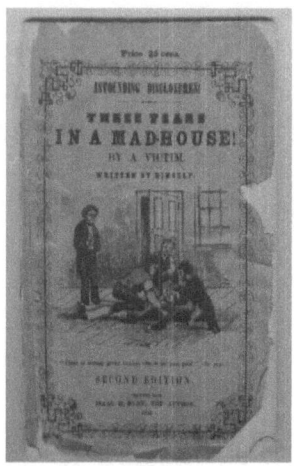

Dr. Ray would later be exonerated of Hunt's allegations, but damage was done to the hospital and the movement as a whole.

Of the experience Hunt writes,

> *On the 21ˢᵗ of September 1844, I was admitted to the Maine Insane Hospital, a wild maniac.... The first assay they made was to have me swallow some pills...I refused but was forced to submit to the treatment ... These compounds had the affect to destroy my bodily health for the residue of my earthly existence..."*
>
> *I now call upon you, Dr. Isaac Ray, the author of a work known to the scientific world as "Medical Jurisprudence for Insanity," a man whose reputation stands in the very front ranks of philanthropy and science in America and Europe. You whose reputation for morality, benevolence and humanity has no superior, and which you have obtained wholly by writing that book and your other scientific writings.*
>
> *You have said to me that no secret of the Institution was ever reveled in the work, you that left me as an incurable maniac and would have murdered me had you even supposed that I could ever come forth to the world again clothed as I now am in the armor of reason and sanity.*

To you and to the public I say, here are a few more disclosers
of your deeds of darkness…

Hunt's allegations were not completely without merit. Many treatments used by early clinicians would be considered barbaric by today's standards.

The terrible draught Hunt spoke of and the pills, may have been the "Blue Pill," a collection of herbs mixed with conium that was often chased by an alcoholic beverage.

With no watchdog groups such as the FDA, hospitals often had their own apothecary, creating mixtures of chemical and herbal remedies that had untested efficacy and unknown side effects.

Hard cases were dealt with using the more powerful and addictive agents such as opium, cocaine, and morphine. Some patients were sedated to the point where they were down for weeks, doctors hoping their extended repose might bring relief and maybe even a cure.

The Maine Insane Hospital also employed the "Bath of Surprise," where a patient was held underwater untill nearly drowned with the water as cold as possible. It was felt that the shock, or "excitement," caused would cool a mania or perk up a depressed patient.

When restraint was needed, patients were strapped into beds or shacked in kicks and cuffs to prevent doing harm to themselves or their attendants. Although Ray was against any kind of abuse, he was forced to meet unruly situations with appropriate measures.

But methods of treatment and restraint taking place outside the hospital were even more bizarre.

Ray noted this in his year end-report of 1842:

Some of the patients before coming to us have been bled,
purged, blistered, setoned, mecurialized while others have been
subjected to repeated course of Thomosonia treatment. Two under
our care the present year were severely scourged, one by the friends
who mistook her insanity for ill temper.

By the time Hunt's allegations made print, Ray had moved on to Butler State Hospital in Rhode Island. Ray had summarily dismissed the accusations, calling Hunt only partially cured at the time of his release.

In the October 24, 1850 edition of the Kennebec Journal, a report on Hunt's allegations was made that publicly exonerated Knapp, Ray, and others:

> *By the politeness of Dr. Simonton, we have been furnished with a copy of the report of the legislative committee appointed last summer to investigate the charge of Isaac Hunt and others against the offices of the above named institution. We have not room to give any extended synopsis of the report. A brief notice of some of the more important points of the evidence and the decision of the committee upon them must suffice. As to Mr. Hunt's personal case, the committee are unanimous of the opinion that he was not abused, as he alleges, "By improper medical treatment."*
>
> *…After a careful examination of the report we are of the opinion that there is but little ground for any serious charges against the officers of the institution, unless a want of proper vigilance over the conduct of the attendants may be considered as such. But the evidence goes to show that whenever abuse came to the knowledge of the officer, the attendants committing them have been discharged.*
>
> *An occasional investigation, however, into the affairs of the Hospital will prove a wholesome safeguard against possible abuse. The nature of the institution and of the authority vested in the officers is such as to render improper treatment and abuse of the patients easy to be committed, and difficult of detection.*

Until his death in 1881, Isaac Ray continued the debate over what deemed a person insane, and not responsible for his or her actions, and what punishment, if any, should suit the crime.

The argument was stretched to the limit by both sides, including Robert Ingersol's view to include a reprieve for all criminals. Ingersol wrote:

> *"Is it not true that the criminal is a natural product and that society unconsciously produces these children of vice? Can we not safely take another step and say the criminal is a victim as the diseased and deformed and insane are victims?*
>
> *We do not think to punish a man because he is affected with disease, our desire is to find a cure. We send him not to the*

*penitentiary but to the hospital or to an asylum. We do this be-
cause we recognize the fact the disease is naturally produced, that
it is inherited from parents or the result of uncurious negligence
or it may be recklessness, but instead of punishing we pity.*

*If there are diseases of the mind, of the brain, as there are
diseases of the body, and if these diseases of the mind, these defor-
mities of the brain, produce and mercenarily produce what we
call vice, why should we punish he criminal and pity those who
are physically diseased? (3)*

Dr. Ray looked forward to the day when he believed that medical
science would solve the mysteries of the mind.

But he was convinced that cures for insanity could only be achieved
if the whole of society assumed the responsibility for the care and the
treatment of those afflicted.

* CHAPTER TEN *

A DAY IN THE LIFE

*"No, it's not bad here. Not as good as home,
but better than the convent."*

Constance Fisher, 1956

O N JUNE 26, 1954, Constance Fisher was discharged from Superior Court observation and readmitted to the Augusta State Hospital as a prisoner/patient.

Although she had been acquitted of a multiple murder charge, she was now a ward of the mental health commissioner and was considered a criminally insane person.

The action had the feel of a prison sentence. She was to be committed to a locked ward and given only those privileges which could be given to patients contained in locked wards.

She could not leave the hospital under any circumstances and would be under constant surveillance and supervision. She would have no outside privileges, and not be allowed the usual patient privileges of educational classes, entertainments, and occupational therapy.

She was told of the verdict by Dr. Richard Marquadt who said the hospital must submit to the conditions, rules, and regulations as prescribed by the court.

Constance accepted the verdict without misgivings, saying, "Oh, I understand. I know that rules have to be obeyed. I will keep busy and do everything I can to help people. I know this can't go on forever."

She asked Dr. Marquadt how long she might be committed to the hospital: one year, five, ten, … life?

"As long as I know it isn't as long as ten years, I can stand it all right. I will still be a young woman," she said.

As far as the restrictions went, they could be lifted or re-defined at the call of Dr. Sleeper.

The small city in which Constance Fisher was now a member was to the general public a place of mystery and dread. Unfortunately, it was exactly such an erroneous perception that prevented Mrs. Fisher from seeking help there in the first place.

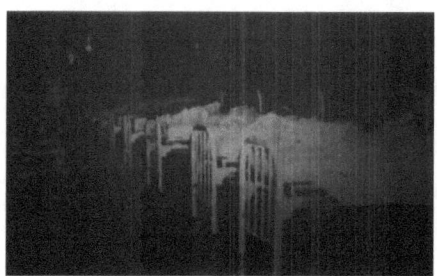

No Vacancy.
Beds line the hallway of the Augusta State Hospital in 1949.
Lack of staff and overcrowding plagued the Sleeper
era at the Augusta State Hospital.

Dr. Sleeper worked hard to eliminate the negative misconceptions and outright lies that dogged the hospital. He made the hospital as transparent as he could to the public, and the agencies set up to regulate its practice.

He used the local newspaper to advertise events happening at the hospital. He submitted feature stories on patients who had recovered and returned to their normal routine of living.

Once a year he held a "Hospital Day," where the whole complex was open to the public to come and see for themselves. If they did not like what they saw, they were encouraged to become part of the solution instead of part of the problem.

Dr. Sleeper sought the aid of area churches and service organizations like the Grey Ladies, to bring their talents and caring to the hospital. Local high schools were invited to perform plays and musical performances before staff and patients. Professional people were recruited to teach classes or a trade to patients interested in broadening their horizons.

Sleeper encouraged visitations from family members and had an adopt-a-patient letter writing campaign for those whose families had forsaken them, or died off.

From this effort to encourage community involvement flowed a greater understanding about the needs of the mentally ill. It also created a bridgework for patients to obtain jobs, friends and places to stay after they were released or out on trial visits.

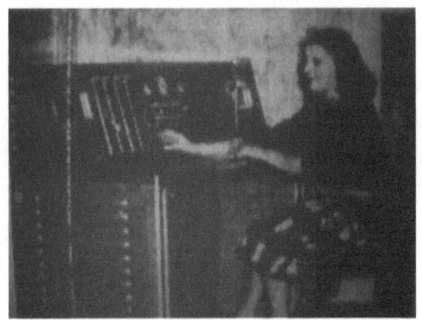

Switchboard Operator?
No, it's a DJ.
Dr. Sleeper believed in the power of music to calm,
refresh, and inspire patients. He had music piped into
every ward and featured patient request shows.

Dr. Sleeper believed in the importance of physical fitness and employed a recreation director who organized team sports and trips to the YMCA for swimming, basketball, and bowling.

He created a literary arm for the hospital, a monthly, patient- written newsletter called *THE OUTLOOK* of which he was the managing editor.

THE OUTLOOK was a compilation of activities and news items from each patient ward, written by its own correspondent. It was a virtual window into the day to day life of patients and staff at the hospital.

In every issue was a two inch block titled, "YES, THERE IS A

CURE," that gave monthly statistics on those who had been let out on trial visits or had been discharged from the hospital.

Although the terms of her confinement prohibited Constance from leaving the hospital grounds, it was not so for other patients.

A patient reporter for *THE OUTLOOK* gives the following report of an outing at Bangs Beach:

> *During the morning, despite a biting wind out of the west, 19 of the "Harvesters" donned bathing suits and charged for the beach but pulled up quickly as the screams of the leaders came down wind. The lake felt cold at first brush but several brave ones forged ahead and half the followers dipped an expectant pedal digit.*
>
> *On the beach there was ball tossing and record playing until dinner which was served Indian style with the warm earth serving as chair and table. Orchestral background music issued from an album of Elvis "The Pelvis" Presley's latest Rock Or Roll (yes, we mean Rock or Roll). Either you're with it and rock, or roll and grimace in pain at the hic coughing tremolo of the Rock'n roll Messiah.*

In what became a public relations bonanza, Dr. Sleeper invited newspaper reporter Brooks Hamilton to the hospital and allowed him unrestricted access, day or night.

The access given Hamilton was unprecedented. The willingness on the part of Sleeper to be completely transparent proved that he did not have much to hide. In fact, Dr. Sleeper felt that he had a lot to show; that the facility was worth every penny invested into it by the legislature and private benefactors.

Hamilton's pass to enter the hospital any place at any time allowed him to make observations about how patients were treated, how effectively the facility operated, and what life was like on the inside.

Hamilton's findings became part of a six-part series that was run by the Daily Kennebec Journal. (1)

Hamilton wrote:

> *What's it like inside an insane hospital? The bugaboo of popular superstition, even today, has that sort of institution pegged*

as a jail-like set of dungeons right out of Dante's Inferno and full of babbling, violent, Napoleons, murderers, Jack the Ripper artists...

People still call the hospital attendant a guard and see him as a King Kong, continually wrestling with violent patients...Even the highly skilled and trained psychiatrist is usually looked upon with some misgivings by his fellow citizen. It is commonly said he has "gotten to be as crazy as the inmates."

Going to the hospital is not a trip anyone looks forward to. Going to a mental hospital is probably worse because for generations we looked on insane as a personal blight on one's reputation; and we haven't gotten entirely over it yet.

What Hamilton found came as a revelation to him and undoubtedly many of his readers. One of his first observations was that many of the patients appeared just as normal as his colleagues in the newsroom.

And he was amazed to discover how prevalent mental illness was, striking one out of every four Mainers at some point in their lives. "The great likelihood is that you or a family member might someday need treatment at a facility like this," he wrote.

Hamilton said that his visits left him with a sense of gratitude that such a hospital existed, especially for the many who could not afford a private institution or the services of a psychiatrist.

Hamilton spent the better part of two weeks touring the complex. He made his way through the medical and surgical facilities, the administration offices, and the wards that held almost 2000 patients.

He visited every ward, and interviewed staff and patients alike. He was most interested to see how the patients were treated, and to note their quality of care and quality of life.

Hamilton witnessed that treatment offered at the hospital was fitted for the entire person, not just the mind. He found an entire medical center there complete with surgeons, optometrists, dentists, cardiologists, gynecologists, neurologists, and chaplains, who worked along with the psychiatrist to restore the patient to health, body, mind and spirit.

In interviewing patients Hamilton noted that many appeared to carry on normally, while others, whom Hamilton described as "hopeless unfortunates," were resigned to custodial care with their cures "beyond the reach of the medicine of this time."

Hamilton learned that the majority of the population was considered curable and that with the right treatment and sufficient time, they could return to a productive place in society.

He found that the hospitals greatest challenge however, was not in finding successful treatment options. The therapeutic model of caring for the whole person was time honored and successful, almost without question.

He found that Dr. Sleeper's greatest challenge was garnering enough support from the state legislators to properly care for his increasing case load of patients.

Sleeper vigorously campaigned for more housing to correct the chronic overcrowding, and he needed the ability to pay and attract competent staff.

Further complicating the matter was the hospital now becoming a destination for the homeless, drug addict, alcoholic, and anyone else in need of food and shelter.

The additional burden ate into Sleeper's budget and attached issues that neither he or his staff were equipped to handle.

Hamilton then turned his attention outside to the grounds. It was the spring of the year when Hamilton conducted his interviews, and the horticulture that decorated the campus was in full bloom and fragrance.

Sleeper believed in the Kirkbride philosophy of having well maintained buildings and attractive landscapes. He believed that first impressions and appearance was more important than most realized.

Hamilton found the campus adorned with a variety of fruit trees, flowers of diverse colors and fragrance, shrubs of many varieties, precisely mowed lawns, and cultivated fields. The air and the grounds were full of life and exuded health, just like the original designers had meant them to be.

Hamilton commented on the aesthetics of the hospital and the work being done on the hospital grounds. He noted the cleanliness of the hospital inside and out, and the constant activity of painters, repairmen, and husbandmen to keep it that way. He spoke favorably of the good tasting nutritious food offered in the cafeteria, almost all of it baked fresh, or a product of the live stock and gardens on campus.

Hamilton's report stated that the campus had grown from the original Stone Building and farmland to include 600 acres and a complex of 59 separate buildings. Also included was a working farm, with a large barn and several out-buildings, that contained equipment and stored meat, poultry and produce. Hamilton counted 300 acres of pasture land, 147 head of cattle, and 90 acres for growing fruit and vegetables. The poultry plant had 3,000 birds, and 1000 laying hens.

Dr. Sleeper believed that keeping the hands full and mind busy was one of the quickest roads to recovery and one that brought a measure of self-esteem and satisfaction. Clinical trials confirmed that when a patient is not engaged in some constructive, satisfying activity, personality assets rapidly deteriorate.

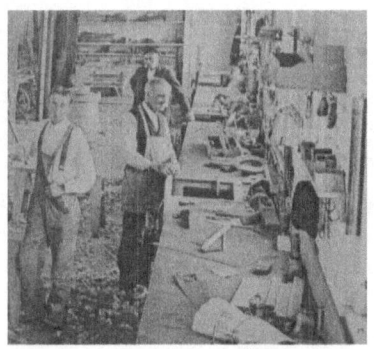

Woodworking shop at the Augusta State Hospital, c. 1905. Making and repairing furniture was considered therapeutic for patients and gave them a skill to take back to the community when released.

Hamilton calculated that the cost of food, housing, medical services, education, entertainment and other services at the hospital to be $1.67 per patient, per day. He concurred with Dr. Sleeper that the same package of services rendered on the outside would be many times that amount and untouchable to most Mainers.

And for over 95% of the patients, the hospital and its various offerings were free.

The niceties offered, that some called spurious, Sleeper argued were critical to the recovery of patients. Hamilton commented on one of the latest additions, a beauty salon.

When the word got out a few months ago that a full scale beauty parlor was being installed at the Augusta State Hospital for the use of women patients, the tax payer yells could be heard from York to Aroostook.

"We'll have to put a stop to that-imagine furnishing a beauty parlor for those inmates out of taxpayers money!" was one (legislators) comment. Sleeper's comment was, "Our patients are human just like you are. We don't want to give these patients humane treatment like that just to look good. We do it because this is the way to start many of them on the road to recovery."

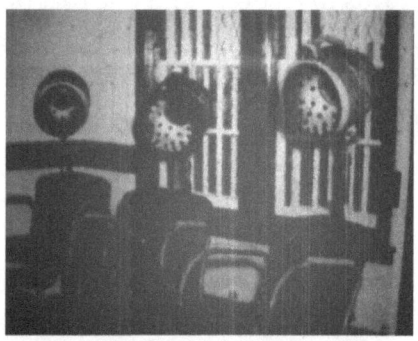

Beauty salon at the hospital, c. 1950
Increased self-esteem was considered essential,
not frivolous, to patients in recovery.

Brooks Hamilton's writings, at least for a while, helped to change the public perception of what really went on at the Augusta State Hospital. No longer did it appear to be the "nut house" that people made fun of and avoided at all costs.

The articles by Hamilton led the Guy Gannet Publishing Company, which owned a chain of Maine newspapers, to write the following editorial:

Long regarded as the skeleton in any family closet, the position of the mentally sick person is a difficult one even in modern times. We like to think we live in a more advanced age than those of former times. But two factors stand out as most general concerning public feeling today towards the mentally ill, showing that our thinking about them is hardly as advanced as our thinking about new automobiles, radios, and refrigerators.

A reporter for this newspaper was given a set of keys and allowed to visit any part of the hospital at any time for a period of several weeks, made a similar finding, and his series of articles has created wide interest in the hospital's problems.

Not only must the public exert influence on the legislature, it must also take an active interest in the hospital. The most striking discovery the Journal reporter made was not any condition inside the hospital, but the almost barbarous attitude of the public towards mental institutions.

He found that a large percentage of the patients never have visitors from one year to the next. While overworked doctors and attendants try to cure as many as possible, a visit from a friend or relative is considered to be one of the best aids to recovery.

It looks as if the legislature will do its part by providing enough room and sufficient staff to care for these sick people. How about you- do you plan to do your part?
(2)

The editorial also raised the question of why, with almost half the nation's hospital beds taken up by mental patients, far more money is spent in research to find a cure for cancer?

The editorial left it up to the reader to judge if the hospital had enough money, equipment, and staff to provide the kind of care expected if they or a close family member were to go there as a patient.

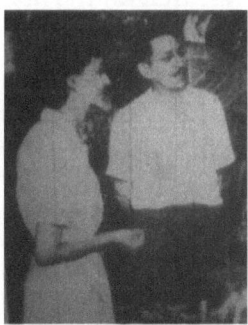

Dr. Francis Sleeper in 1949.
It was said that Sleeper knew the names of every patient in the hospital as he greeted them on his rounds. In a sad and ironic twist of fate, he became one of them later on in life.

When Constance Fisher entered the hospital in 1954, the institution had perhaps reached its zenith in regards to treatment options and programs offered. It was likened to a city in a city, with a population that exceeded several area towns. Combining patients, staff, employees, and visitors, the population could reach 3,000 persons on any given day.

And there was no doubt that Dr. Francis Sleeper was mayor of said city. A mustached man of diminutive stature, he ran the institution after the model of Dr. Ray and other moralists. Under his charge, the hospital was cutting edge, humane, and transparent. A man of faith and vision, his sentiments are best summed up in his benediction for the year 1954 as expressed in *THE OUTLOOK.*

Superintendent's message

> *At this Christmas season we pray that the leaders of the nations may be granted such wisdom that all people may once again enjoy the happiness of peace on earth, good will toward men.*
> *May it be granted that the healing efforts of the employees and staff of the Augusta State Hospital be blessed with increasing success that more of our patients may return to happy living with friends and relatives.*

A Maine native and graduate of Bowdoin College, and Boston University Medical School, Sleeper interned at the Worcester State Hospital where he did extensive research on the body's metabolism and its relationship to mental health.

His study focused on chemical change triggered by glands as a cause of mental illness, bucking the trend that most mental health problems developed in childhood and were caused by poor parenting or trauma.

He came to the Augusta State Hospital in 1949, looking to add to the repertoire of treatments and resurrect some old ones, like Electro Convulsive Therapy and Insulin Shock Therapy which had fallen out of favor with the prior superintendent.

Dr. Sleeper imposed strict rules prohibiting abuse of patients in any form. He did not allow any constraints or seclusion except by written order of a doctor and counter-approved by him.

A visionary, Dr. Sleeper believed that ultimately psychiatric care should be established in every community. In the mid 1950's he began a traveling clinic that sent doctors from town to town offering psychiatric care and counseling. Unfortunately, the project was disbanded for lack of funding.

In 1958, he established a pilot Community Mental Health Clinic in Lewiston which Sleeper believed to be the most efficient manner in providing care. He advocated having a local resource to treat short-term situations while keeping the state hospitals in Augusta and Bangor for the chronic and dangerously mentally ill.

He opened several half-way houses in the Augusta area as well as having a "night hospital" where patients on the verge of recovery could work during the day and go back to the hospital at night.

Dr. Sleeper probably did more to put a kinder face on the institution than any of his predecessors. Although his main goal was to get patients well enough to return home, he endeavored to make their stay at the hospital, educational, enriching, and even enjoyable.

It is both ironic and sad that later on in life Dr. Sleeper would himself battle mental illness. He developed Parkinson's disease, which forced his retirement from the Augusta State Hospital in 1963. He would on occasion have psychotic episodes, perhaps a side effect from the medications he was taking.

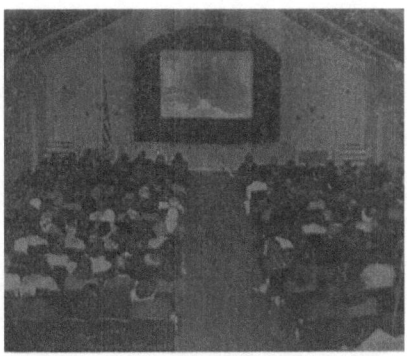

Patients enjoy a movie at the Augusta State Hospital, about 1950.

For Constance Fisher, life at the institution could best be summed in the words of Charles Dickens: "It was the best of times, it was the worst of times."

Here, due to the notoriety of her crime, she was the center of attention and curiosity. And that lay in the hospital's best interest. The reputation of the hospital could rise astronomically should she be treated successfully, perhaps enough to even be released.

Constance found the attention, not only from the hospital staff but from her family, to be healing. The feelings of neglect and disconnect from her foster mother that had buffeted her throughout childhood were atoned for here. And whatever differences she and Carl might have had, well, their absence from each other only made their love fonder.

Constance would spend most of her stay in Middle Stone, a low maintenance, unlocked ward where most of the higher functioning patients lived.

She lived in a dormitory-style room with few amenities, although she made her room homey with things brought from Carl and her family.

In many respects, it was an improvement over the conditions at Snow Pond or even the apartment in Waterville. All the essentials of living were provided at no cost, as well as opportunities for intellectual development, recreation and friendship.

She was among the fortunate to have visitors, sometimes several times a week, and always at least once a week from Carl. She received packages from her mother, with food clothing, money stamps and other essentials. She could attend Mass in the chapel daily, and struck up a lasting relationship with Father Lemire.

Constance easily became acclimated to and even thrived under the scheduled, structured, and unburdened life at the Augusta State Hospital.

From letters written home, it appeared that she took full advantage of the opportunity and worked hard toward the goal of getting well and getting back to Carl.

One of her letters to Carl gives a snapshot of the social life there:

> *…Yes, we had a good party right after supper we all gathered in Martha's room we talked a while then we started in on the eats. Boy oh boy, I've gained 3 or 4 pounds and Martha has gained 15 pounds since she has been here.*
>
> *We have a lot of fun and it helps the others… We are still going ahead with our club we call it the Mental Delinquents Club. We have 15 members so far and more want to join. We discuss our*

*problems, our inferior complexes and we are using the Alcoholics
Prayer as our motto and have drawn up a few rules.*

   *At the last party I got them to playing charades, each one gets
up and acts out a song title and the others have to guess it. It was
a lot of fun and everybody enjoyed it...*

THE OUTLOOK records that Constance participated in several activities during her first stay at the hospital. She played on the women's softball team, participated in the yearly ministerial show and several drama events. She took courses in ballet, crafts, and participated in group therapy sessions. She was one of the first to participate in a new offering at the hospital; psycho-drama, where patient's acted out their feelings and frustrations.

She was also a contributor to *THE OUTLOOK,* that featured several of her poems.

For the most part, Constance Fisher was considered a model patient. She mixed well with patients and staff, readily engaged therapy, and eventually became a candidate for release.

But as Dr. Ray had warned nearly a century earlier, if patients are pushed out the door prematurely, the results can be, and often are, tragic...

* CHAPTER ELEVEN *

RELEASE

"The right to restrain an insane person of his liberty is found in that great law of humanity which makes it necessary to confine those whose going at large would be dangerous to themselves or others."

Lemuel Shaw, 1845

MAY 6, 1959, WAS the day that Constance Fisher had longed for, hoped for, and prayed for. She had finally secured a district court hearing that might enable her release from the hospital.

Her fate would now rest in the hands of the honorable Judge Richard Dubord, the same man who had represented Mrs. Fisher at her murder arraignment. He now had the authority to keep her at the institution or set her free.

At 10:00 a.m. Mrs. Fisher was taken by police cruiser and transported the short distance from the Augusta State Hospital to the Kennebec County Courthouse. It was the first time she had left the institution in five years.

Representing Mrs. Fisher was F. Harold Dubord, the judge's son, who was accompanied by Dr. Sleeper and Dr. Marquardt, who would be called upon to testify in her behalf. Carl Fisher would also be called to testify.

And Constance Fisher would be allowed to make her own case that she was now fit to return to society, and that she was no longer a danger to herself or others.

After a brief hearing, a meeting of council was held in the chambers of Judge Dubord, where Dubord went over the options at his disposal:

- He could deny the request outright.
- He could deny the request but recommend that Mrs. Fisher be allowed a series of trial visits to see how she fared away from the hospital.
- He could grant a release, but mandate regular visits to the hospital to insure a relapse would not occur.
- He could exercise the option that would guarantee that the tragedy never be repeated: have Mrs. Fisher sterilized, and then released.

Since 1925, there had been legislation on the books that entitled state of Maine run agencies to perform sterilizations. It was done in mass at the Maine Industrial School for Girls in Hallowell, an institution designed to "re-train destitute and delinquent girls."

Part of the "re-training" was to forever prevent them from passing on their predisposition to delinquent behavior to another generation.

And there was an economic argument pushing sterilization. Why not just eliminate another generation that might be a life-long burden to taxpayers, either through welfare or the corrections system.

The initiative was known as Eugenics, or the science of improving the human condition through controlled breeding. It was an offshoot of Darwin's theory of the survival of the fittest and was first promoted by Darwin's cousin, Francis Galton.

It gained acceptance at the federal level of the United States in 1927, and elicited this response from Supreme Court Justice Oliver Wendell Holmes, Jr.:

It is better for all the world, if instead of waiting to execute degenerate offspring for crime...society prevent those who are manifestly unfit, from continuing their kind. (1)

By the 1930's, the movement had gained an almost global acceptance. In the United States, 33 states had laws on the books to sterilize
any woman deemed dangerous to society.

But after the atrocities of Hitler's Germany; its extermination of
undesired groups and the supposed creation of a master race, Eugenics
quickly fell out of favor.

In the case of Constance Fisher however, such a drastic measure
might have been favorable.

It would have guaranteed that Mrs. Fisher never destroy her children again, and if seen as punitive, might make her release a little more
palatable to the public.

But it was Dr. Sleeper's firm recommendation that the court give
Mrs. Fisher a pardon and his opinion prevailed.

After the council closed chambers, the Fishers were told that Constance would be released under the provision of section 120, of Maine
state law, that says that:

> ... *if anyone is found innocent by reason of mental defect of
> any crime, then rehabilitated and cured, said person could return
> to society without recrimination if found to not be a threat to
> oneself or the community.*

The piece of legislation dated back to March 17, 1821, enacted
shortly after Maine became a state. The original provision reads as follows:

> *Be it enacted by the senate and house of representatives, in
> legislative assembly, that whenever any person who may have been
> arrested and in custody or in prison to answer for any crime or
> crimes, offence, or offences, before the supreme judicial court shall
> be acquitted thereof by the jury or trials or shall not be indicted
> by the Grand Jury, by reason of insanity or mental derangement
> so such person, and the discharge, or going at large of such person
> shall be deemed by the same court to be dangerous to the safety of
> the citizens or to the peace of the state, the said court be, and herby
> is authorized and empowered to commit such person to prison,
> there to be detained till he or she be restored to his or her right
> mind, or otherwise deliver by due course of law.*

Commit such person to prison? It would be another 20 years before a treatment facility would be built to distinguish a prisoner from a patient.

At about noon, Judge Dubord signed an order of discharge, which was confirmed by Judge Marden. The order was then delivered to Carl who returned to the hospital the next day to pick up his wife and her belongings.

Incredibly, Constance Fisher, who confessed to the murder of her three children, was now free with no strings attached!

Before leaving the hospital she was seen by Dr. Sleeper for the last time. She was given a charge that she would be expected to conduct herself beyond reproach and that she could be picked up and returned by any legal authority if evidence of misconduct or disease appeared .

A tearful Constance Fisher shook her head in agreement and promised Dr. Sleeper that she would conduct herself in the best manner possible, and contact him immediately should she need further help. After a brief embrace, Constance Fisher was now free to return home.

On Friday, May 7, Carl Fisher drove to the front steps of the Stone Building. He watched as his wife walked down the long granite steps with a suitcase and a few boxes. Attendants loaded the remainder of her possessions in the back of the Chevy truck he had borrowed from his father-in-law, Warren Marcoux.

It all seemed like a dream, but a dream much different than the nightmare that brought her to the Augusta State Hospital a couple of light years ago.

For Constance Fisher, it was nothing short of a miracle. A miracle that she had her health back. A miracle that her husband wanted to try again at their marriage. A miracle that someone who had performed one of society's most heinous acts, had a clean slate and a fresh start.

What a difference a day makes. The night before Constance had spent alone in a small room with a single barred window. Tonight she would sleep with Carl for the first time in five years, two months, and 29 days.

And her return would not be to the primitive setting of the cabin on Snow Pond or the cramped quarters of their second-story Waterville flat.

Carl had built her a dream house, the one they always longed for but were financially unable to attain. And not just a house but a farm, with a stream that ran through he middle of it.

The farm came with acres of fields that they could plant and raise animals on. It would be just like it was during the happiest days of her life, when she lived with Silvier and Rose on the Riverside Farm.

And she and Carl could start a family again, although it had been strongly recommended that Constance be sterilized.

Perhaps that was Dr. Sleepers going away present to her. It was his ultimate vote of confidence that whatever had troubled Constance Fisher before would not come back again. But Dr. Francis Sleeper was not always so sure...

Φ Φ Φ Φ Φ Φ Φ Φ Φ Φ Φ Φ Φ Φ Φ Φ Φ

By 1955, CONSTANCE FISHER had shown enough improvement that she was transferred from Middle Stone to Middle Tyson, where she had more freedom and liberties to attend classes, entertainments, and other activities.

She was also allowed to do occupational therapy, working in the employees' dinning hall, a job she had requested. She insisted the she was no longer having delusions, mood swings, or hallucinations.

And she was no longer having those awful nightmares where the children would appear to her crying and asking "Why Mummy, why did you kill us?"

Constance had also become aware that her return to health might have another positive consequence. Carl had been told by their attorney, F. Harold Dubord, that if deemed cured by her doctors, she had a legal right to petition for release.

And Carl was making moves towards that end. With the proceeds left from selling the cottage on Snow Pond, he had recently bought a plot of land in Fairfield Center. He had been advised that buying the property might be a good sign that a secure and comfortable place was being prepared for Mrs. Fisher at an appeals hearing.

In July of 1955, a formal request for hearing was made to Dr. Sleeper, who after calling special council with his staff, returned his verdict to Judge Richard Dubord.

It read:

Dear Judge Dubord:

I am sure that Mr. Fisher has been acting in good faith when he says he feels his wife has shown a great improvement. Superficially this is true. On the other hand, I assume that you are asking me for satisfactory proof that the discharge will not endanger the peace and safety of the community. This I cannot give…

Under the circumstances, considering the seriousness of her crime and the very definite possibility of a relapse as indicated by abnormal pathology in her projection tests, I am in no position at this time to suggest to any Justice of any Superior Court that this patient, in my opinion will not endanger the peace and safety of the community.

This patient has been subjected to insulin therapy. The most recent information regarding insulin therapy for the psychosis from which she suffers is that these patients tend to relapse. Therefore I feel in duty bound, both in Mrs. Fisher's interests and those of the community, not to recommend her release at this time.

Respectfully yours,
Francis H. Sleeper, M.D.

Dr. Marquardt weighed in with the following observation:

The writer has recently been told by one of the employees that she overhead Mrs. Fisher state she is not going to stay in this place very much longer, that her husband has ways of contacting a lawyer to get her out of here before fall.

It has been noted by the writer and by others that Mrs. Fisher, when in public, seems unusually happy and gay, singing, whistling, chatting, and the writer has had several patients, who suffer from conflicts which almost led to similar overt acts as those which were completed by Mrs. Fisher, state that they could not understand how a person seeming to be of sound mind, could be so happy and care-free after having done what she did.

It is the writer's opinion that Mrs. Fisher has displayed some more of a sociopath behavior pattern since her staff conference was held on June second, than she did prior to that.

Constance Fisher took the denial in stride. She told Dr. Marquadt that even though she was denied appeal, she felt physically, emotionally and mentally well and fully capable of taking care of the present and future, and that if given the opportunity would prove to society that she was fully recovered from her illness.

In mid-1957, the same procedure was again initiated by Carl Fisher. As bound by law, Dr. Sleeper was once again forced to bring together Mrs. Fisher's doctors and others to make a determination on her fitness to return to society. Their rendering is given in the following summation:

July 3, 1957

Dr. Saunders:
I notice that there were no tears for the tragedy, no sobs for the slaughter, only tears for Connie, concerns for Connie, "I am sure I would never hurt myself or my husband." That egocentric trend is still present. I do not think she is well enough for anyone to guarantee to a judge that this woman will not follow the same behavior when the going gets tough.

Dr. Canal:
I don't think so either. I don't know enough about the patient, but I doubt in my mind as to the Schizophrenia, I don't know what it is. I don't think she should go, I think she is unpredictable.

Dr. Moore:
I don't think I would want to go before a judge and say she is well.

Dr. Lighthart:
I would not want to commit myself to a judge. I do think that she sill does not display affect. She has been studying up on what has been told to her that is lacking in her personality, and she has tried to fill it in.

Dr. Jeanne Hecht:
No, she should not go.

Dr. Sergeeff:
No

Dr. Senenkyj:
No

Rev. Whittier:
No

Father Lemire:
I don't think she should go. If she cannot go on a short trial visit, then my answer is no.

Mr. Covatta:
No, she is still homicidal.

Mr. Kawliche:
No

Mr. Streitfeld:
No

Dr. Sleeper:
The staff is unanimous in the opinion that it would not be proper to issue a statement to the court to the effect that this patient is no longer a menace to herself or to society; therefore, no such statement will be made at this time.

Constance Fisher would have to wait another year before the appeals process could again be put into effect. Her privileges at the hospital were expanded, and she began taking courses in ballet and ceramics.

She told Dr. Sleeper that she was reasonably contented at the institution and had gained a much broader perspective on life and what it takes to be healthy mentally and emotionally. She said that life at the hospital was better than in the Convent but, of course, she would be much happier in her own home.

And she believed that she was both morally and legally acquitted for her murders.

This idea presented a dilemma for her doctors. Not wanting to burden Mrs. Fisher, or Carl for that matter, with the overwhelming guilt of the crime, they had to set the record straight.

Dr. Marquardt wrote the following after a conversation with Mrs. Fisher on July 8, 1957

> ... Mrs. Fisher made a number of statements which were alluded to either by a lawyer, doctor or priest, that said she would not have to be here very long, and that she was morally and legally not responsible. This was of course, meant in a way quite different from the way the writer tried to fix it in the patients mind.
>
> The writer tried to impress the patient again, that if the same acts were committed by a so-called sane person which were committed by her, a so-called insane person, were treated equally in Maine, the law had not decided in her favor by the phrase not guilty by reason of insanity, the sentence for taking human lives most certainly would be more than five and most usually considered at times up to life.

Carl's interpretation of the crimes was also disconcerting.

> What was more surprising was Mr. Fisher's reaction to this conference. A few days after he came to the writer's office and tremblingly announced that he had consulted a lawyer regarding his wife's release...
>
> It soon became evident that Mr. Fisher, much less than Mrs. Fisher, seems not to realize the seriousness of the crime against humanity which has been committed. He, somewhat like the patient, still reasons that she was declared not guilty, and he therefore sees no reason why she could not be discharged and that they could get their trailer and move to California.
>
> The writer tried as effectively as he could to show Mr. Fisher that Mrs. Fisher was declared not guilty be reason of insanity by the superior court of Maine. He still was unable to accept that and said, "It's a funny thing, in other states women do things like that and much worse and they are going scott free."

On July 28, 1958, Constance Fisher was once again interviewed to determine her fitness to return to society. A staff meeting was held with Doctors Sleeper, Marquardt, Saunders and Canal being present. They noted there was no evidence of any psychosis for almost three years now, and that Constance had adapted extremely well to life at the institution.

The question of whether or not the patient should be recommended for release to a Superior Court Justice was debated before answered in the negative by Dr. Saunders and Dr. Marquardt.

Dr. Canal and Dr. Sleeper were of the opinion that she was displaying no symptoms of mental illness at this time. They agreed that Mrs. Fisher had performed well in the interviews but Dr. Sleeper pointed out that, "She has a superior intelligence and is very adroit in presenting the best aspects of her personality to the staff."

But Dr. Marquardt observed that Carl was "highly nervous," and had recently sought help from Dr. Sleeper and himself on how to calm this condition and wondered if he should be put on some kind of medication.

Also waving a red flag was social worker George Greeley. Greeley had recently conducted an interview with Carl at his farm in Fairfield Center. He noted that Mr. Fisher, "appears rather depressed and apathetic. He reveals little information, did not smile, and responded slowly."

Greeley reported that while the home was being updated it still was in need of major renovation and had two rooms still unfinished. The farm had acres that could be cultivated but was in need of the purchase of a tractor. Other expenses included a mortgage payment of $40 per month, taxes set at $83, house insurance at $32, and his car payment.

These of course, were not insurmountable amounts, but Carl Fisher had no savings. And he had just been laid off from his job and had no idea when he would be recalled by his employer. Given the fact that financial hardship was given as a catalyst to Mrs. Fisher's first onset of illness, it was surely a cause for concern.

Greeley's final observation was harrowing:

> *The worker couldn't help but think, as he sat in the kitchen and was looking through the open door directly at the bathtub,*

as the door was opened to the bathroom which adjoins to the kitchen.

Those familiar with the case will know that if Mrs. Fisher were in this environment, and like most of the housewives, spent her time in the kitchen, she would have a constant reminder of the unpleasantness..."

Because the opinion of the doctors was not unanimous, it was decided there would be no recommendation made for her release.

"There is no way at this time, to predict what Mrs. Fisher might or might not do if she were placed in similar frustrating situations which precipitated the murder of her three children," was the professional opinion written to Carl Fisher's lawyer, F. Harold Dubord.

It was explained to Carl Fisher, in a letter dated July 29, 1958, from Dr. Sleeper :

Dear Mr. Fisher,

I am writing this letter to inform you this in accordance with my promise to you and Mrs. Fisher, I have today reviewed the case of Mrs. Constance Fisher, your wife, together with three other doctors, all psychiatrists.

The four of us were in partial agreement that Mrs. Fisher has adjusted herself satisfactorily to the hospital routine. They could not agree that they or I can make the unqualified statement to any person that Mrs. Fisher no longer constitutes a menace to herself and/or society at this time. Neither consent, nor reconsideration for the presentation of her case before the Superior Court will be made at this time.

If you are not satisfied with this decision, you may apply for a Writ of habeas Corpus if you so desire. If you are not satisfied that the Staff and I have acted in accordance with our best judgment, you may request that Mrs. Fisher's case be presented before me again at the expiration of 12 months, which could be as early as July or August, 1959.

Dr. Francis Sleeper.

It was Carl who informed his wife that once again her appeal had been turned down, and that she would be in the hospital at least another year before he could even start the process again. A letter to her mother, intercepted by the hospital, said this about the rejection :

> *"Hi"*
>
> *Just a little note to let you know that I am alive and kicking- and kicking is the word for it. Carl said he saw Jackie and Stubby and told them the verdict so you probably know by now.*
>
> *I just can't see their reason and they haven't had the thought- fulness to even see me and talk it over. Honestly, they are so au- tocratic they get my dander up. After all we're not children, they should talk things over more intelligently. I think it is only up to them to say whether I am sane or not and I know that I am and have been for a year or more.*
>
> *I'm going to have a good talk with Richard Dubord and get a few things ironed out. I think I should have seen more of him. They did not level with me on the legal aspect as Richard told them to Carl. We shall see. I'm not taking this lying down...*

From a clinical standpoint, it was apparent that Mrs. Fisher was too great a risk to release back into the community. Too risky to even be considered for a trial visit, a next step that was often given to patients transitioning from the hospital back home.

In 1957, staff at the hospital had voted down this option feeling that Constance was still not stable and possibly a flight risk, as she had been talking about moving to Florida or buying a trailer and driving to California.

But now a new pressure was mounting on Dr. Sleeper to release Constance Fisher.

A revolutionary movement was growing across America that was rapidly gaining the support of ideologues, politicians, and activists. It was called Deinstituionalization and its goal was to scale down the large mental hospitals in favor of community clinics that would treat, release, and ease patients back into the community. It's silver bullet was seen in the potential of a new generation of anti-psychotic drugs.

Deinstituionalization received its original launch in 1955 when the Joint Commission on Mental Health decided that the federal gov- ernment should get more involved in the state run mental hospitals. It concluded through surveys that state- institutions were holding almost 500,000 Americans, and that many of the hospitals were plagued by scandal and abuse.

And the institutions were seen as financial liabilities, and growing ones, as the population of the mentally ill was increasing in step with the national population.

Maine became one of the first states in America to put precept into practice. In 1958, "Operation Out" began to hand pick candidates from the Augusta State Hospital to be released outright back into the community.

Who knows what discussions might have taken place behind the closed doors between Dr. Sleeper, Maine governor Clinton Clausen, and representatives from the Eisenhower administration. If Operation Out could prove a successful model, perhaps the rest of the nation would quickly follow.

And sitting in a single room on the second floor of the Tyson Building at the Augusta State Hospital was a poster child for the new movement: Constance Margaret Fisher.

After all, her story had made national, even international news. What if, in a reasonably short space of time, Mrs. Fisher could be rehabilitated to the point that she was safe to readmit into society, even safe enough to have more children?

A stretch? Perhaps. But something of momentous imperative took place in the winter months of 1958 that caused Dr. Francis Sleeper to reconsider his position, ignore established protocol, and make a fatal decision.

In a direct contradiction to his letter of July 29, 1958, Dr. Sleeper decided to take up the Fisher case again in March of 1959.

On April 6, 1959, he issued this communication to Carl Fisher:

Dear Mr. Fisher:

I am writing you this letter to inform you that on March 31, 1959 I made the recommendation to the presiding Justice of the Kennebec County Superior Court, Augusta, Maine, that on March 30, 1959, Mrs. Constance Fisher, your wife, was examined by the entire Medical Staff, and that it was the finding of the staff that Mrs. Fisher does not at this time present any positive psychotic signs or symptoms of psychotic behavior.

In accordance with the provision of Chapter 27, section 120, of the Revised Statutes of 1954, Mrs. Fisher was presented to the Presiding Justice for confiscation. On April, 3, 1959, Justice Harold C. Marden of the Superior Court of the State of Maine informed me that he is willing to consider the petition of Mrs. Constance Fisher.

It seems that it is now up to you to present the petition to the Court, and to acquaint yourself with the manner in which you should proceed from now on. It is possible that the Clerk of Courts, upon your request, will be able to assist you regarding the correct manner of procedure.

Dr. Francis Sleeper

In a strange and confusing turn of events, Constance Fisher, who had repeatedly been denied even trial visits, and on three occasions considered by her doctors unfit for release, was now on a fast track to freedom.

Φ Φ Φ Φ Φ Φ Φ Φ Φ Φ Φ Φ Φ Φ Φ Φ Φ Φ

ON OCTOBER 26, 1959, the hospital initiated a final check up on Constance Fisher, this time at her home in Fairfield Center. The interview was done by social worker George Greeley. Unknown to Mr. Greeley, Constance was once again pregnant.

His report read:

She greeted writer very warmly, smiled and invited him into the house. We chatted about patients she knows at ASH. Mr. Fisher had been in the bathroom and now joined us, shook hands with the worker and asked him about his luck in hunting. As usual his face was practically expressionless, except for a constant depressed look. This is the way he has always appeared to worker.

Mrs. Fisher seemed much more cheerful than when she was

in the hospital. The house appeared very neat and clean as did the grounds. Mrs. Fisher had no complaints and there was nothing unusual in her behavior, appearance or conversation. The only noticeable change was her teeth; all of her front teeth appear to be half-decayed."

Even without notification by the hospital, news of Constance Fisher's release spread quickly into the community.

And not everyone applauded the decision. The Waterville Sentinel ran a tardy, brief statement on the release but refused to editorialize it.

The residents of Fairfield, while hesitant, seemed willing to give Mrs. Fisher another chance. The mood of the community was forgiving but apprehensive. Some questioned that if she had a relapse, could she commit this crime against somebody else's children?

But most vocal in his concern was Dr. Edgar J. Smith who wrote an angry letter back to the Augusta State Hospital when Mrs. Fisher came to see him during the pregnancy of her fourth child, Kathleen:

> *...I have been taking care of Mrs. Fisher since early in her pregnancy. She came to my office stating that she had been going to another local physician who had referred her to me for obstetrical care. However, no information concerning her general health had been forthcoming from the referring physician.*
>
> *...With realization of the patient's past history and in retrospect, it is noted that I have never seen nor talked to the patients husband which is consistent of a usual pregnancy, and is not unusual. But in this case at least a little unusual. Moreover, I do feel that the fact that she never came during regular office hours, presented herself at the latter part of the day or on a Sunday morning is in the light of her history, perhaps a little unusual...*
>
> *I was rather upset of learning of her past history in the round-about method in which I did. On hearing of it I called Dr. Sleeper, superintendent of the Augusta State Hospital. He tells me the story was in all the newspapers which I am in agreement. In speaking to Dr. Sleeper he assured me that in his opinion the patient is perfectly all right and should be treated as a normal pregnancy...*
>
> *She was committed for life to the Augusta State Hospital, Criminal Division, because of the previous murder of her three*

children. In Dr. Sleepers opinion she is cured of the illness which precipitated the act and he feels she will have no further difficulty in this respect…

On hearing of the past history, I contacted the patient and asked her why she had not told me what had gone on before. She stated very matter of factly that this had transpired in the past and she thought it was of no importance in the present episode.

As far as I am concerned, the patient undoubtedly needs obstetrical care which we are willing to provide. Despite Dr. Sleeper's advice to treat her normally, I am still somewhat in doubt as to how I shall handle her postpartum. She will be admitted here when she is in active labor, will be observed and watched closely, particularly in reference to her actions in and about the hospital.

Following delivery, I am not sure as to what will transpire. I do believe, however that I will follow Dr. Robertson's advice. Dr. Robertson and I read Dr. Sleeper's abstract over together. Dr. Robertson is of the opinion that she should be seen at least once a week for psychiatric evaluation for some 3 months. This I feel, is not within my province. I am a general practitioner of medicine and have the usual general practitioners knowledge of psychiatry.

It is my intent following delivery to send Mrs. Fisher voluntarily to see Dr. Sleeper at the state hospital and to let him handle any post partum psychiatric developments which may occur, as he knows more of her in this respect and a qualified psychiatrist is not immediately available in this area.

Dr. Sleeper wrote back in response on March 24, 1960:

Dear Dr. Smith,

This is one of the most pitiful cases that we have experienced…

Of course the hospital is entirely willing to do anything it can to be of help in the final and complete rehabilitation of the patient. As I told you over the telephone, we are not possessed of a crystal ball, we cannot guarantee that everything will go well with Mrs. Fisher for the rest of her natural life.

Under the statutes, when I believe that a patient no longer constitutes a danger to self and others, it is my duty to release this patient. This was done legally and properly before a superior court justice and on the testimony of Dr. Marquardt and myself, both of whom have had an excess of thirty years experience in psychiatry.

I am most unhappy that Mrs. Fisher did not tell you from the start that she had been discharged from this institution. The circumstance of her admission here were very sad. She was actively psychotic at the time and she had been for two or three weeks prior to the tragedy...

We have no way of forcing Mrs. Fisher to have psychiatric help; legally we have no right to lay a finger on her or to insist on her coming down here; however if she wants to come or if she wants to see any other qualified psychiatrist we will be happy to cooperate to the limit...

Frankly, I do not anticipate any such difficulty however, we are not infallible and it is within the realm of possibility although I consider it highly improbable. If she should develop a post partum psychosis it would probably be a reactivation of her old basic schizophrenic reaction pattern and she should be promptly returned to the hospital on a precept from a superior court justice. The statement of a single doctor would be sufficient.

Very truly yours,
FRANCIS H. SLEEPR, M.D.

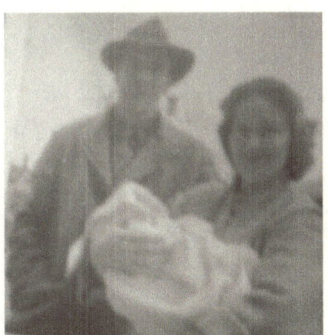

Carl, Constance, and Kathleen Fisher, 1960.
Not everyone was pleased with the Fisher's decision to start another family.

In January of 1960, Constance Fisher delivered her fourth child, Kathleen. And soon the family would increase to three with the birth of Michael Jon in 1962, and Natalie Rose in 1965.

Although almost as cloistered as they were on Snow Pond, from all appearances the Fisher's had a normal, happy life, and the farm was a haven to the Fisher children and their cousins.

And Aunt Peggy became a favorite to her nieces and nephews. Her sister, Jacqueline Chamberlain later said that her children were very fond of Constance. They thought the farm was the perfect place to live with the goats and the kittens and all the toys. They even commented that if "mommy ever went away, we would like to go out and stay with Aunt Peggy."

Carl was doing well at his job at the railroad and had a little carpentry business on the side. Constance seemed happy and fulfilled in her life as a housewife and a mother. And although American society was caught in an unprecedented turbulence in the early and mid 1960's, all appeared amazingly stable at the Fisher household.

But as the family grew, Dr. Smith continued to sound an alarm. A post-partum trigger doesn't always follow the birth of a first or second child. It can lie latent through multiple pregnancies before manifesting itself.

In 1965, while treating Mrs. Fisher after the birth of Natalie Rose, Dr. Smith apparently detected trouble and tried to put the hospital on alert. An inter-departmental memorandum dated December 14, 1965 to Dr. Walter Rohm, stated:

> Social worker telephoned Dr. Edgar J. Smith Fairfield 453-6343.
> Dr. Smith stated that he wished to discuss the case of Mrs. Fisher with Dr. Patterson, had some "Fine Points to go over with the doctor."
> He claimed he has treated Mrs. Fisher since her discharge from A.S.H. but gave no information on present state of her health. When worker suggested a visit to Dr. Smith's office for current information, was told, "will discuss only with doctor."

Constance Fisher would later confess that she had spells of depression during the time between her hospitalizations. But she never told anyone for fear that she might have to return to the Augusta State Hospital and then, "who would take care of the children?"

But when Constance could no longer hide her depression after the birth of Natalie Rose, Carl insisted she go back to the hospital. Constance objected however, arguing that she could work her way out of it.

And she failed to tell her husband that she was hearing voices again, and getting homicidal ideas. And all too soon, the ideas would once again turn into deadly actions.

* CHAPTER TWELVE *

DEJA VU

*"If only I could have held out for a few more days, the depression
would have passed and this would not have happened…"*

Constance Fisher, July 1966

Thursday, June 30, 1966, 4:30 a.m.

THE ALARM WENT OFF as usual on a bright, sunny day in central
Maine. Temperatures hovered around 70 degrees, and it was promising to be one of those blue sky, great-to-be-alive, days so common to
a Maine summer.

Carl Fisher got up at 4:30, early enough to get ready for his day as
a box car builder at Central Maine Railroad, about a ten-minute drive
from his home on the Ohio Hill Road in Fairfield Center.

He had chores to do around his 60-acre farm; chickens to feed, and
other animals and pets to care for. He checked in on the vegetable and
flower gardens as this promised to be a good growing day.

Carl set the screens in the doors and windows of his two- story bun-
galow, and then skimmed the headline of the morning newspaper that
had just landed in his yard.

Soon, his children would be arising, looking forward to the best part of the day; the undivided attention they received from their father before he left for work.

Carl Fisher is now a middle-aged man, 46 to be exact. His hair is graying, his face thinning. His long prominent nose accentuates his gentle green eyes.

His frame is slender, that of a hardworking Mainer who has struggled to make ends meet. Somewhat of an introvert, he stays at arms length from his neighbors and had no real close friends. The nearest house is almost a quarter mile away.

His countenance is somewhat sad and shy, the product of life experiences that would have crushed a lesser man.

He is the kind of man you would like to have as your military comrade, one who would take a bullet or smother a grenade to save your life. He is faithful to a fault, his word is his bond.

Born on Christmas day, 1920, Carl Merrill Fisher was brought up in the poverty of the Great Depression and spent four years in the armed services fighting in World War II. He is the embodiment of what one journalist called the "greatest generation."

As Carl started breakfast, the baby, Natalie Rose, now almost nine months, began to cry. The noise awakened Constance, who had been home from the hospital for just a few days. Carl had taken the last three days off to make sure that the house was perfect, and that everything would be comfortable for her return.

Constance Fisher arose to get Carl a cup of coffee, and to assure her husband that she felt fine and had in fact enjoyed a good night's sleep for the first time in weeks.

Constance had not been feeling well for some time, since perhaps March. It had been a long, cold winter, one that drags on and makes many Mainers "snow birds" in their retreat to a warmer climate.

But there was no such reprieve for Constance. She commiserated with her sister Jackie that she was feeling depressed again, although nothing like before. Jackie commented that she had not been feeling too well either.

"I feel like a statue full of cracks that would break if anyone struck it" Jackie Chamberlain said.

"With me it is more like being made out of springs. I am either wound up tight or loose," said Constance.

They spoke of a mutual friend who was going through a post-partum depression after the birth of her daughter. Constance expressed empathy for the friend saying, "When you feel like that, you just can't tell anybody about it."

One gloomy day in late March, Carl came home from work to find his wife in bed, where she had stayed most of the day. The baby, blonde and blue-eyed Natalie Rose, had been taken care of but six-year old Kathy, and four-year old Michael Jon were running wild.

There were coloring books and toys scattered through out the house and the beds in their rooms pulled together and used as trampolines. Somehow they had managed to make dinner for themselves without disturbing their mother.

For most of her adult life Constance was given to blue moods or funks. They would usually follow her menstrual period. Most were of a short duration, but this one lingered long enough so that Carl sought professional help. He made an appointment to see Dr. Price Kirkpatrick, a psychiatrist at Seton Hospital in Waterville. Dr. Kirkpatrick was the one who had set up the community mental health center in Waterville, the newest trend in the treatment of mental illness.

After seeing Dr. Kirkpatrick, Constance was prescribed a new medication regimen. It was Kirkpatrick's recommendation that she be hospitalized while trying out the new medications but Carl objected.

"She is still nursing now and I don't know if she will want to go... I asked her and she didn't want to go," Carl Fisher said. Kirkpatrick asked Mr. Fisher if he could stay with her a few days while she adjusted to the medication, to which he willingly agreed.

The regimen brought immediate relief.

"I wish I had known about them years ago," Constance commented. "They take the weight of the world off my shoulders."

The cost of the medicines however, between $15- $20 a week, was a lot of money in the Fisher household. It became a source of concern to the frugal Constance who handled the couples finances.

Carl would lovingly affirm they were worth any price if they made her feel well. And they did, for a while.

In early June, Carl Fisher returned home after work to find that his wife had, once again, not even gotten out of bed. It was like before, the baby was taken care of but the other children were left to run wild. Carl found remnants of peanut butter sandwiches and toys strewn around the house.

He wasted no time in contacting Dr. Kirkpatrick who recommended that Constance be admitted to the hospital as a patient in his care. Distressed, fearful for herself and her family, Constance went willingly this time.

On the night of June 21, 1966, Constance Fisher was admitted to Seton Hospital, medicated, and put under observation. She complained of being depressed, and not being able to think clearly. She admitted that the care of the children, her oldest in particular, was wearing her down. She had only recently stopped nursing the baby, who was now cutting teeth and fussy.

As always, Carl was there to take up the slack. For much of the past two months he had cared for Constance, cleaned and picked up the house, and continued working towards making an upstairs bedroom for Kathleen. But the missed time from work was accumulating and putting his job in jeopardy.

From June 21 to June 25, Constance was a patient at Seton Hospital. The timing of the hospitalization canceled the family plans for a week together at their cottage on Snow Pond.

Carl, in particular, had been looking forward to the family vacation. A few years before, he had purchased the lot, and built a small wood framed building. Recently he had added running water, stove, and refrigerator.

The family loved spending time there, enjoying water sports, fishing, boating and the children investigating the wonders of nature.

The camp had primarily been used as a weekend getaway, but the family was excited about spending a full week there now that summer was in full bloom and the days were getting longer and hotter.

And Carl was also looking forward to doing something special for Constance. June 29 would be their 20th wedding anniversary. To those who knew, it was nothing short of a miracle the marriage had survived so long.

But the plans were put on hold due to the hospitalization. Constance had daily visits from Carl, who now took his vacation week to care for the children. Every day, Carl would bring his wife tape recorded messages from the children and Constance would record a response in reply.

Carl and the children embarked upon a major spring clean so that everything would be nice, fresh and friendly for Mummy's return. Carl had recently added a new washing machine and electric dryer to ease her work load. He also installed a humidifier to help her chronic sinus problem.

Having Mummy in the hospital was a new experience for the children. The mental health problems Constance had suffered in the past were kept there. They were never talked about among family or friends and certainly not to the children.

On Saturday June 25, 1966, Dr. Price Kirkpatrick made perhaps the biggest decision of his professional life. He felt the patient had improved enough under "extensive pharmo-therapy" and he deemed further hospitalization unnecessary.

But there was talk among other professionals at the hospital that Constance, given her history, should be sent back to the Augusta State Hospital for observation. It was rumored that Constance herself said that she wasn't ready to go back to care for the children. A nurse was reported to have overheard her saying, "I do not want to go back home, I am afraid to go back home, I am afraid that something terrible might happen."

Her family was also in support of an extended period of treatment to help weather the storm that they knew would pass in time. But Kirkpatrick was adamant. He told Constance that the best thing she could do was to go back home and take care of her family.

Another dissenting voice was Rev. Joseph Brannigan, a parish priest at the Immaculate Heart of Mary Church in Fairfield where Carl, Constance and the three children were members.

Having only recently come to the congregation, Father Brannigan was just getting to know the family and knew nothing of their past.

He had just presided over the baptism of their youngest child, Natalie Rose, and was beginning to make weekly visitation calls to their home.

Rev. Brannigan was concerned about the family's reclusive behavior. Their home was built in the most rural end of town, and down a long road that had no neighboring houses. They had no telephone. He acknowledged it was like the Fishers had almost purposely wanted to be out of sight and out of mind.

Church on Sunday, shopping, and visits to and from family seemed to be the only social venues of interest to the Fishers.

Father Brannigan had struck up a casual relationship with Carl, and found him to be a decent, honorable man. Although he was a man of few words, his expressions often relayed his feelings. And Father Brannigan could tell that Carl was sensing an imminent disaster.

"Carl knew she was in deep trouble," Brannigan recalled later. "And that it would only be a matter of time before the dam broke."

Sometime during the week of June 21, 1966, Father Brannigan made a pastoral visit to see Constance in her room on the third floor of the psychiatric ward at Seton Hospital. He was alarmed at her appearance and somber mood. He confronted Kirkpatrick with his observation, and expressed his concern that she be kept longer.

"It's just a post-partum depression," Dr. Kirkpatrick explained. "It will pass, she will be better off back home with her family and in familiar surroundings."

Neighbor Harvey Wood was also concerned about Constance's seeming premature release. Carl had related to him that her health was bordering on crisis.

And Wood had overheard neighbors saying that Constance was hearing voices through the radio saying that the end of the world was approaching and that she needed to kill the children and do it fast.

Wood was surprised that she was not re-committed to the Augusta State Hospital. He questioned Kirkpatrick's judgment saying that even the average lay person would know just by talking to her that she was on shaky ground.

But in the end, Price Kirkpatrick opted to release Constance Fisher to the care of her husband with the strict recommendation that she continue her medication regime.

A copy of Constance Fisher's release from Thayer Hospital reveals the following:

> *Mrs. Fisher was admitted for the treatment of a post partum*
> *depression with a hesitant and concerned feeling that there might*
> *be a psychotic element to this illness but, upon closer observation*

and with respect to the way she responded to medication, there was no sign of a previous postpartum psychosis in this illness.

Mrs. Fisher, who was very depressed and sleepless, distraught, concerned about herself in admission, responded very rapidly to the antidepressant drug Nardil and the tranquilizing drug Mellaril and, in the course of a very short hospitalization, regained her sense of well being, her normal sleep pattern, her interest in her surroundings and, at the time of discharge today, 6/25/66, she is smiling, pleasant, more than eager to be home and take care of the responsibility of her home and children.

Final Diagnosis : Postpartum depressive reaction
Condition on Discharge: Markedly improved.
Prognosis: Excellent.

Dr. Kirkpatrick told Carl that the medications would make her a little drowsy but would soon wear off, and that bed rest would be a good idea. Carl took the following three days off from work, to make sure there would be a smooth transition. He later said that Constance seemed improved, very improved, and went about her house work and care of the children.

On the morning of June 30, after spending his week vacation caring for his wife, Carl Fisher kissed Constance and his children goodbye, grabbed his lunch pail and the keys to his Land Rover truck.

He turned before closing the screen door, once again inquiring as to whether Constance felt well enough for him to return to work. A smile and a nod, told him things were okay.

But Carl Fisher had his doubts and suspicions...

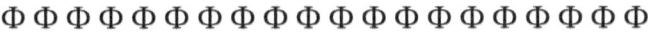

Thursday, June 30, 1966 4:00 pm.

IT WAS A ROUTINE day back at the rail yard and Carl was happy to be back at work. After the whistle, he ran a few errands around town before heading home.

He drove down the long dirt-coated driveway, noticing but paying little attention that the children's toys, always prominent in the driveway on sunny days, were still indoors.

He pulled the vehicle behind the house and headed towards the barn to inspect the hen's eggs before making his way to the front door.

The strange silence was the first thing to arouse his attention. Usually, the children were all out to greet him by now, followed by Constance with a glass of lemonade or something else cold to drink. But now there was nothing but the whispering wind stirring up dust from the driveway.

A dreadful anticipation flooded Carl's mind. Every sordid image of the time before flashed before him. His heart pounded as he began to mop the sweet from his forehead.

Carl Fisher went around to the front door only to find it locked. It was a screen door and it was locked from the inside, latched by an eye hook. He hollered in but there was no reply. He ran to the master bedroom window, looked inside, but saw nothing.

Back around to the front he summoned his strength and courage, tore off the screen door, and entered the house. He ran straight ahead, down the hallway to the only bathroom in the two-story structure. There, he found his baby, Natalie Rose, naked, face down, and dead in an inch and a half of water.

The dirty rings on the side of the bathtub told Carl Fisher the fate of his other children as well.

He then bolted out of the house and drove up to the house of Harvey Wood who was putting away his tools for the day outside his front yard.

Wood greeted his frenzied neighbor, learned of the tragedy and agreed to accompany him back to the house. But first he placed a phone call to Fred Gould, chief of police in Fairfield and then to Father Brannigan. Together, they drove back down into Fisher's driveway and waited for assistance to arrive.

Father Brannigan was the first to arrive and did his best to console one now inconsolable.

Brannigan had been hearing confessions that afternoon when the parish secretary frantically paged him saying, "Father, they need you immediately up to the Fisher residence." By now Brannigan had become familiar with the tragic past of the couple who were now his spiritual responsibility.

Chief Gould arrived within a couple of minutes and the two men entered the house, while Carl waited outside his parked vehicle, leaning up against the driver door for support.

Followed by Father Brannigan, Officer Gould entered the house through the rear door. He proceeded through the rear porch and then into the kitchen located on the south-east corner of the house. Just to his right, in a room off the kitchen was the bathroom that contained a small bathtub.

Entering the room Gould found the lifeless body of Natalie Rose Fisher. Her head was just above the drain, which was partially plugged by her curly blonde hair and a wash cloth. A dirty ring on the side of the tub indicated that the water was once about eight inches deep.

Knowing that there could be three other occupants in the house, either dead or alive, Gould proceeded down from the kitchen to the living room.

There lying on the couch covered in a blanket, was the body of Michael Jon Fisher. Completely naked, his small frame was cold to the touch and Gould noticed a frothy foam around his lips. There were no visible marks on his body, leading Gould to conclude that this child had also died by drowning.

Gould's journey through what was now a house of horrors was only half done. He moved down the corridor to the bedroom on the north-east side and found another child, covered in a blanket and completely naked. Gould identified the body as being that of Kathleen Fisher.

After moments that seemed like eternity, Father Brannigan appeared at the door and delivered the words Carl Fisher anticipated but dreaded to hear. In a quivering voice he shouted "They are all gone, they are all dead!"

At that, Brannigan stepped back inside to give the children their last rites.

Seeing the ambulance and the police cruisers, neighbor Ansley Wilson ran over to the house to see if he could give any assistance. As he attempted to comfort his trembling friend and neighbor, he heard Carl Fisher say,

"I just wish she could have left me just one of them."

Back inside the house, Captain Gould made his way to the master bed room. There he found Constance Fisher. She was lying on her bed covered with a blanket, unconscious. He peeled back the bedding and could see no visible signs of injury, but detected that she was still breathing.

His call to have an ambulance waiting was, at least for the moment, fortuitous. He noted some stab wounds where Mrs. Fisher had apparently tried to injure herself with a kitchen knife.

Lying at Mrs. Fisher's side was a pistol that shot .22 caliber pellets and the knife. On the bed stand were the empty bottles of three prescription medicines. The prescriptions, Nardil, Mellarill, and Thorazine, taken together in that amount, should have been enough to kill a horse.

On the table, a suicide note was left to her husband. Scratched in pencil on the back of a greeting card she wrote:

Dear Carl,

   I hope you understand, it's the only way I could be sure they would go to heaven. I can't bring them up right. I've already had such a bad influence on them. They could never grow up right. I' m sorry, so terribly sorry it turned out this way. O Carl if I could only tell you how terrible it is to feel this way...

The parking lot was now filling up with policemen, detectives, and media. Father Brannigan took Carl up to the Wilson house where they called and waited for his sister Helen Zimba to arrive.

He was given a sedative to help him calm down and later a tranquillizer to help him sleep.

He could only hope this was all just a terrible nightmare, only reminiscent of the time before. Maybe in the morning he would wake up and everything would be all right...

Never again would Carl Fisher return to the scene of the tragedy. But the property would continue to be plagued by tragedy. The next residents, the Raymond family, would lose two of their children outside at play in a freak accident.

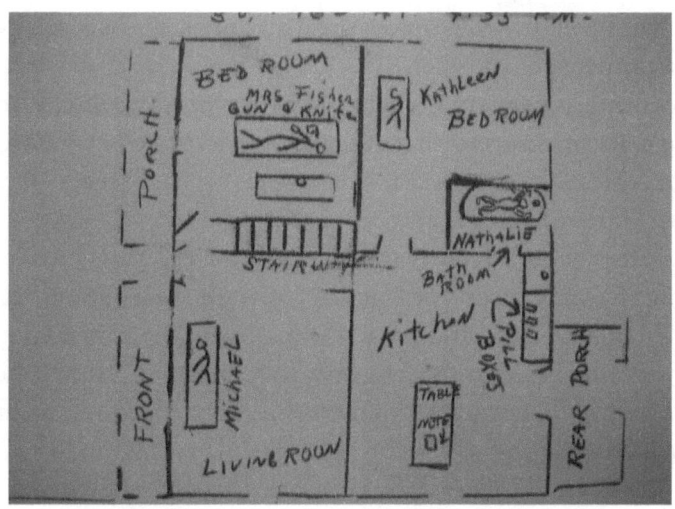

**Sketch of the murder scene drawn by Police Chief
Frederick Gould at 4:35 pm, June 30, 1966.**

Thursday, June 30, 1966, 8:00 pm

AFTER GATHERING EVIDENCE FROM the crime scene, police were given the unenviable task of putting the Fisher children into body bags to be delivered to the morgue. Last to leave, Lewry Brothers Ambulance Service transported Constance Fisher to nearby Thayer Hospital.

A brief examination in the emergency room found her to be semiconscious, with a small reddish mark on her chest.

She had shot herself with the pistol, and Dr. Joseph Heibel, the emergency room physician, removed several of the bb pellets from her abdomen. He also had her stomach pumped, finding the remains of the undigested capsules she had used in trying to overdose.

Mrs. Fisher was then taken to room 302 in the east wing of the hospital and put under guard.

Meanwhile, four floors beneath, the bodies of her three children were autopsied by Dr. Maurice Philbrick. He found no marks on the bodies to represent a struggle. No puncture wounds or bruises, no bullet holes or trauma. His conclusion was simple and straightforward: the children had been drowned to death. Also conclusive was the perpetrator of the crime; their mother.

Twelve miles away at his father's house in Oakland, Carl Fisher arose in a state of emotion that can only be described as indescribable.

He had awakened to find it was not just a bad dream. It was déjà vu. It was March, 8, 1954, all over again.

Carl Fisher would later blame himself for the tragedy, wondering why he did not pick up on the signs of Constance's deteriorating condition earlier. Maybe he could have taken a proactive approach and simply had her committed to the Augusta State Hospital. Maybe he should have followed his gut and not allowed Kirkpatrick to release her until she was ready. One thing was for sure, he did not blame his wife.

"She never would have done this if she wasn't so sick," he told police.

Back at Thayer Hospital, the drama continued to unfold. In the morgue, Dr. Philbrick pulled white sheets over the lifeless bodies of the three Fisher children at 10 p.m. His final atonomical diagnosis read: "asphyxiation by drowning."

Lying on a bed in her single room, Constance Fisher was very much alive and alone with her thoughts. Outside her door, Chief Gould and representatives from the District Attorney's office, Richard Cohen and John Benoit arrived to discuss their next move.

Benoit came at the request of assistant attorney general Cohen, who had been alerted of the tragedy by his wife, Susan. He had just come home after arbitrating a murder case and had collapsed on the couch when his nap was interrupted by a phone call about the Fisher tragedy. He phoned Benoit as much for moral support as legal opinion.

The autopsy was already in progress when the men were escorted into the morgue. What they observed was so disturbing that Cohen had to walk out.

The youngest child, Natalie Rose, lie on the examiners table naked from the waist up and clothed in only shorts. Half of her face had been removed. Her tiny body, the innocent victim of an evil disease, lay stiff and cold.

Officer Bodman stood in the hallway outside Mrs. Fishers room as a security guard when Dr. Philbrick arrived and gave his verdict that the children had been drowned to death, evidently by Mrs. Fisher.

They would soon be joined by Captain Albert Drost of the Waterville Police Department, and Sheriff Henderson, who were given the okay by Dr. Hiebel to begin an interrogation.

The Waterville Police Department later issued a summation of the interview:

> *We were informed by Dr. Joseph Heibel who was treating Mrs. Constance Fisher that Mrs. Fisher was awake and that she was coherent. Mrs. Fisher was in the new wing of the 3rd floor, Room 302, that is a private room.*
>
> *Captain Drost and Sheriff Henderson entered the room. Mrs. Fisher was laying in bed with her eyes closed. Captain Drost called her by name, "Mrs. Constance Fisher" and she replied, "Yes."*
>
> *Captain Drost introduced himself to Mrs. Fisher and then proceeded to inform her of her rights, that she need not say anything that would involve her in any way in any offence, and if she did say anything that whatever she did say could be used against her. She replied, "I know."*
>
> *Mrs. Fisher was further advised that she could have an attorney now before any questions were asked and that if she was not able to get one a lawyer would be provided for her to be present at the hospital with her during questioning. Mrs. Fisher replied, "I don't want one."*
>
> *Mrs. Fisher was again advised that if she was not feeling well enough, no questions would be asked and she replied, "No, I am all right." She again was asked if she wanted to answer questions but that she did not have to, and again she replied, "I understand."*
>
> *Mrs. Fisher was asked by Captain Drost if she knew him and she replied, "Yes I do, you talked to me about the first three children, the same thing as now," and she further stated, "You were very nice to me then like you are now."*
>
> *Mrs. Fisher was asked by Captain Drost if she knew what happened to her last three children and she replied that she did and that "they are now in heaven."*
>
> *Mrs. Fisher was asked what happened to these children and she replied, "I drowned them all." She was asked where and she replied, "In my house," asked where and she replied "In my bath-*

tub." She further stated that she filled the tub but did not change the water between drownings.

Mrs. Fisher was asked which child was first and Mrs. Fisher replied that Michael was first, Kathleen second and Natalie was third. Captain Drost asked Mrs. Fisher what time it was today when it happened and she replied in the morning, that she told the children they were going to have baths, and when asked if the children had breakfast she replied, "some."

Mrs. Fisher stated that they did not fight or scratch her, she stated she told them "It will only hurt for a minute," and that she held each child's head underwater for a little while until each was still.

Mrs. Fisher was asked if she was sorry about what she had done to the children and she replied, "No, I am not, the children would have had a hard life ahead of them, and now they are in heaven."

Mrs. Fisher was asked if she was going to do anything to her husband and she replied, "No, well, I could not figure out a way to do it." Mrs. Fisher was asked what she planned to do with the gun and knife found in her bed and she replied, "I was going to shoot myself and the gun did not work, and I was going to use the knife but I fell asleep."

Mrs. Fisher was asked why she drowned her children and when she first thought about drowning them. Mrs. Fisher stated that she thought about drowning the children for "some time," asked why and she replied "they were always hollering and shouting and I could not take care of the baby."

Mrs. Fisher was also asked if she received help from anyone during these times and she stated she had been to Dr. Kirkpatrick, but that he did not help her.

Mrs. Fisher was asked once again if she was sorry that she had killed her children. She replied in a matter of fact tone, "No, I am not. They would have had a hard life, they are better off now, better off dead."

On Friday night, June 30, 1966, after completing an interview with Captain Drost and Sheriff Gould, Constance Fisher was arrested and taken to a facility for women in Skowhegan and then taken the Kennebec County Jail where she was held without bail until her arraignment.

On Saturday, July 1, 1966, as Constance Fisher slept in a jail cell in Augusta, her children Kathleen Louise, Michael Jon, and Natalie Rose, were put to sleep in the ground at St. Francis Catholic Cemetery.

And it was left for Carl Fisher to once again put back the pieces of a shattered life.

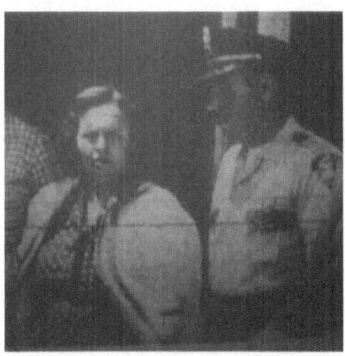

Constance Fisher is escorted from the Somerset count court house by officer Ray Rancourt on July, 5, 1966.

July 5, 1966, Augusta State Hospital 7:00 pm

In Evenlyn Bennett's tenure as a nurse in charge of admission at the Augusta State Hospital, she had seen many bizarre cases, but none came close to this one.

It was her responsibility to do the paper work on patients being admitted and for security and safety reasons she was always accompanied by another nurse and a guard.

First admissions were escorted to a holding area in the Stone Building where they were strip-searched, bathed, and given a medical examination.

At the time, the Augusta State Hospital was the largest psychiatric hospital in the state, and a refuge for the mentally ill, alcoholics, drug users, and those just needing a temporary respite.

Over the years, Mrs. Bennet had been verbally abused, spit on, bitten, and once had her clothing ripped. She observed that mental Illness does not discriminate according to race, religion or social status. She recalled the wife of a prominent politician who came periodically to get electric shock treatments, the only thing that would relieve her cyclical depression.

She told of a doctor's wife who would occasionally show up in full regalia, wearing her mink stole, diamond rings and gold bracelets. She laughed at the story of a waitress who, when her employment waned in the winter months, would check into the hospital until spring.

And there were some who were admitted against their wishes. She recalled the time that a young man, who in the process of being committed, ran down the second story corridor where he jumped head first through a bank of windows. He then fled on foot to the town of Albion, some 20 miles away, and remained in seclusion until his sister called the hospital.

A judge however, declared him to be in his right faculties and decreed that he return home and not back to the hospital. A week later, the man committed suicide.

Mrs. Bennett was at her post when Constance Fisher was escorted into the hospital by the Sheriff Henderson.

It was around 9 p.m. that the phone rang with the sheriffs department saying that they had arrested Mrs. Fisher on the charge of murder and they were bringing her to the hospital for observation.

In her admission notes, Bennett stated that Mrs. Fisher was calm, and cooperative upon arrival, and that she submitted readily to the regular routine of paper work and evaluation.

Her ledger read:

7/5 1966 9:20 pm

> *Brought to Augusta State Hospital by Sheriff of Somerset County and two matrons for examination, interviewed by Dr. Hirshberger....*
> *Was told by Dr. Hirshberger that every word said could be used against her, also that she did not have to tell anything that she didn't want to tell. Dr. Hirshberger asked,*
> *"Are your tired?"*
> *"A little."*
> *Where did you come from?*

"Skowhegan, I was in Augusta this morning and Judge Poulin took me to Skowhegan."

"Do you know why you are here?" "I drowned my three children."

"Were you here before?" "Yes, 12 years ago."

"How long were you here?" "Five years."

"How did you feel after leaving the hospital?"

"I had depressed spells"

"Do you feel sorry for what you did ?"

Yes, I feel sorry, I wonder how I could have thought that way."

She said that she was not taking care of the children properly and that there was no one else to, and that they would be better off in heaven. Mrs. Fisher said that when she was sick her husband wanted to bring her to the state hospital, but that they didn't have anyone to care for the children. She stated that the whole world was in a mess, saying, " hopeless, hopeless, hopeless."

Husband did not know she had suicidal thoughts, was trying not to worry him. Made her feel worse because it was costing him so much money, and it wasn't doing any good. Also stated she had a rough and terrible childhood."

"I felt bad for her I really did", Bennett said later. "I just can't imagine anyone doing what she did. And to have it happen twice…"

On July 6, 1966, Dr. Dimitri Polydefkis, gave the following admission summary after interviewing and observing Mrs. Fisher.

"When interviewed, the patient was dressed in a house robe and appeared in good contact with her surroundings. She admitted with no difficulty to the murder of her three children, and gave "depression" as the reason for her action. She further added that the circumstances of her life in Fairfield were very difficult for her and the demands of her responsibility were getting increasingly greater."

A further admission to the murders was told to John Arthur, a mental health technician, on July 21, 1966

"Mrs. Fisher claimed that she had been quite depressed for

205

two or three months and that she had been on medication but it had not helped very much and it had been changed three times. She said that she had had a mild depression for a while and that it had gotten worse about the time she went to see Dr. Kirkpatrick.

She added at this point she still feels quite suicidal. Mrs. Fisher claimed that whenever she became completely depressed and confused she would sit in a daze and was unable to do the household chores, however her husband was quite sympathetic with her and helped her considerably.

When she becomes depressed no one is able to cheer her up even though her husband does try to do so. Mrs. Fisher said that when she left the hospital seven years ago that she still had some depressions but she was able to control them. At this time they did not overwhelm her completely and she was able to get through these experiences somehow.

However, more recently as the depression became deeper and deeper she became more confused and distant. She described her feeling of confusion as being unable to think straight, to concentrate, or to be able to do things. She describes her feeling as everything just seems so hopeless and that the world seems quite hopeless at times."

It was another four months before Carl Fisher was able to tell his version of what happened. It was in a police interview that was conducted at the Central Maine Power Company building where Carl was working in Waterville, January 11, 1967.

Q. Your full name?

A. Carl Merrill Fisher

Q. And your date of birth, Carl?

A. December 25, 1920

Q . Carl, I'm going to take you back to the incident involving your three children and your wife quite a few weeks ago. I'd like you to tell me exactly what happened on that day, I believe it was on a Thursday. Did you report to work as usual on that day?

A. Yes, I left for work like I did every morning.

Q. What time was it Carl?

A. *About quarter past five.*

Q. *Quarter past five in the morning? This is a day job you have with Central Maine?*

A. *Yeah. Day job.*

Q. *Was there anything at all unusual before you left?*

A. *No. No. I always went in to see her and talk to her before I left and she'd get up to see me off.*

Q. *So everything was normal. Your wife got up on that date and saw you off to work. Nothing unusual at all.*

A. *Didn't seem to be because I wasn't worried.*

Q. *On the Wednesday night Carl, just before that, Carl there was nothing unusual at all?*

A. *No. Not that I can remember.*

Q. *Thursday morning everything seemed normal?*

A. *Yeah. If there was I certainly would not have gone to work.*

Q. *Did she threaten to do any harm to the children?*

A. *Oh, no.*

Q. *Prior to this happening?*

A. *No*

Q. *Nothing was ever said in that regard?*

A. *No. She loved the children.*

Q. *No physical abuse on the children at all previous to this Carl?*

A. *No. No*

Q. *She never touched the children?*

A. *She would, she didn't like it because I would holler at the kids. She was awful easy on them. I would try to make them mind. She hated to say no to them. Of course I'd come home and try to make them mind and she'd feel it a little bit if I would holler too much at them. No, she never hurt the children.*

Q. *Carl, going back again to this Thursday, you left for work as usual. Did you have any inclination at all that anything had happened until you returned home that evening?*

A. *No, I didn't.*

Q. *You don't go home at noon time?*

A. *No.*

Q. *So you tell me exactly what you found, what time you left here, when you arrived home and what your found there.*

A. *Well, I got out of here at three-thirty and I don't exactly know what time I got home, I mean it must have been pretty near four, and I went in the garage and inspect the eggs there we've got two hens, and then I went to go in the house I noticed the screen door was still locked from the inside.*

Q. You noticed the screen door was locked from the inside?

A. Yeah. It was still hooked from the inside so I hollered and I went around to the bedroom window where our bedroom is and I hollered in there and it was very quiet. I was a little worried then and I pulled the screen off.

Q. Off the bedroom window?

A. No. Off the screened door. It was hooked on the inside with and eye hook but I pulled it off and went in the house and looked in the bathtub and saw my baby in there and I knew what had happened.

Q. The youngest one was in the bathtub?

A. Yeah.

Q. Still water in the tub?

A. No. The water had drained, you could see rings on the side. She must have been in there all day. Most of it.

Q. And you left immediately and you went where?

A. I went up to the neighbor's

Q. You indicated, Carl, that the neighbor made the calls to Chief Gould and to the parish priest for you. What did you next do?

A. Well, I went back down to the house and parked my car outside the road there and waited.

Q. You waited outside your home in your car who was the first official to arrive, Carl?

A. Father Brannigan come down first.

Q. Two minutes after the father arrived, Chief Fred Gould arrived?

A. Yes

Q. And then what happened, what took place then?

A. Well, they went in the house.

Q. You stayed outside at this time?

A. Oh, yes.

Q. So you had no idea what they found?

A. Well, Father Brannigan come out and he said they was all gone, they was all dead. He said he gave my wife the Last

Rites and I guess it wasn't until the ambulance come, I don't know if they had a doctor or not, but he hollered out that she was still alive.

Q. *You remained right outside all the time?*

A. *Yes, I didn't go in. So they got an ambulance up there and took her up to the hospital.*

Q. *Is there any other part that you played at all? Did you stay completely out of it?*

A. *I couldn't. Father Brannigan got me to go up to a neighbor. I stayed up there and then he had the doctor give me some pills to take and then my sister came over. She got me to go into her house. I didn't go up near my wife.*

* CHAPTER THIRTEEN *

AFTERMATH

"One of the most bizarre tragedies in New England history."

Boston Herald, July, 1966

O N THE MORNING OF June 30, 1966, everyone's worst fears had become a devastating reality.

The same cast of characters that had triggered the first episode had returned to cause a second.

Financial difficulties, post partum depression, and a fear that the world was spinning out of control, had once again kicked Constance Fisher over the edge.

Within a short period the story was national news, this time sharing headlines with another infamous case, that of Albert Desalvo, the Boston Strangler.

The Boston Sunday Herald of July 10, 1966 ran this assessment:

"Carl Fisher is in seclusion this weekend; his wife, Constance, is in Augusta State Hospital. And their six children are in graves-decorated with wilted geraniums at St. Francis Cemetery.

Law authorities held Mrs. Fisher responsible for the deaths of her six offspring claiming she drowned three of them 12 years ago

*and then repeated the same type of triple murder 10 days ago in
one of the most bizarre tragedies in New England history."*

Something or someone had failed terribly. The medical community?
The judicial system? A fatal breach of personal responsibility? There was
plenty of blame to go around.

Questions as to how and why were being asked across the nation,
as the Fisher murders would become one of the most researched filicides in U.S. history.

Typical was an inquiry by the Massachusetts Department of Mental Health to Dr. William Schumacher, Director of the Bureau of Mental Health and Corrections in Maine:

Dear Doctor Schumacher:

> *A few months ago we read in our local newspapers a report of
> a woman in Maine who was said to have killed her three children
> many years ago while psychotic, and who had subsequently been
> released from the hospital, had given birth to three more children,
> and had just killed those three children as well.*
>
> *We are frequently in the position of having to make recom-
> mendation to the courts or to the Governor regarding the release
> of an individual who has been committed to one of our hospi-
> tals after having been found not guilty of murder by reason of
> insanity.*
>
> *The question always arises, of course, as to whether any such
> individual might repeat the crime for which he had been tried.
> Each such case has to be handled on its merits, and I don't suppose
> that we are ever going to arrive at any useful rules that we can
> apply generally to all such cases.*
>
> *Nevertheless, we wish to learn as much about such cases as
> we can... no doubt we would all benefit if there were some way
> of pooling all of our information on subjects of this kind.*

Many were now willing, perhaps feeling it was their duty, to come
forward to share publicly what they knew.

One of the first to speak was Rev. A. J. Lemire, chaplain at the Augusta State Hospital who had befriended Mrs. Fisher while she was a
patient there.

After her release, Father Lemire would visit on occasion at her Fairfield residence just to stay in touch.

Perhaps Rev. Lemire knew Constance Fisher better than anyone. He was her spiritual advisor. He heard her confessions, and prayers. His role in her life was so critical that Dr. Sleeper had made him a part of her evaluation team.

Rev. Lemire said in a interview dated July 17, 1966, that before the first incident she had sought psychiatric help but had not found any relief for her depression.

He admitted that seven years before, he helped Mrs. Fisher gain her release but even then the hospital staff was not unanimously in favor of it.

Father Lemire said he had seen Mrs. Fisher as a friend and counselor several times since her discharge, the last time a little over a year before the second tragedy.

He said that as far as he knew, and the hospital confirmed, that Mrs. Fisher had received no psychiatric attention from the Augusta State Hospital since her discharge in May of 1959.

But Rev. Lemire said that she was urged upon release to "come running back at the least sign of an upset." Father Lemire admitted that he didn't feel too safe about her release, but didn't feel she should be locked up for life, either.

Rev. Lemire said that a recurrence of such an illness must have given warning signs to any observant person,

"I would expect some sign of it showing up for at least quite a few weeks," he said. It should have been evident to anyone with the least notion of what to look for."

Dr. William E. Schumacher, Director of the State Bureau of Mental Health, questioned how prudent it was to have Mrs. Fisher released to begin with.

He said that the hospital had always erred on the side of caution, and had always taken a conservative approach in releasing forensic patients. He said that only five such patients, including Mrs. Fisher, had been released since the state law had been amended in 1954.

Also weighing in on the tragedy was Dr. Price Kirkpatrick. He told a Portland newspaper that it was probably Mrs. Fisher's negligence in taking her prescribed medicine that led to the tragedy.

Kirkpatrick said that he had prescribed medication for her about a month before the tragedy when it became obvious she was experiencing, " severe depression accompanied by fits of weeping and sleeplessness and mental vagueness." Kirkpatrick said that Mrs. Fisher's disorder was a biochemical ailment that can successfully be eliminated with medication. He noted that four percent of all women undergo hormone changes and they have a variety of effects.

"In Mrs. Fisher's case the effect was the most hideous you could imagine," he told the paper.

He had no doubt that it was a resurrection of the former condition that had resulted in the death of her three other children 12 years ago.

Kirkpatrick affirmed that Mrs. Fisher was perfectly normal and cheerful when he discharged her from the hospital just days before the murders. He said she understood the nature of her illness and that she now had the drugs necessary to curb it.

"Something happened and I don't know what it was," Kirkpatrick said. By our present knowledge, this tragedy just couldn't have happened again if she had taken the drugs properly."

But reporters pointed out that the state hospital doctors apparently didn't diagnose Mrs. Fisher's illness in the same way Dr. Kirkpatrick did. And they didn't prescribe any drugs for her ongoing treatment.

In a letter dated July 18, 1966 Dr. Kirkpatrick summarized his findings for an inquest:

> *I am enclosing my discharge summary from Seton Hospital which reveals that I had become perhaps too quickly optimistic that she had had a pure Depressive Reaction with none of the true psychotic elements of the past, though I had admitted her with a question of a Post Partum Psychosis. Unfortunately my prognosis has not been born out.*
>
> *In health, Mrs. Fisher is a rather attractive, very pleasant conscientious woman, very feminine and very close to her husband. She and her husband appeared to be both exceedingly devoted parents and devoted to each other. There were no schizoid elements in her personally whatsoever when I have observed her in periods of health.*

Mrs. Fisher was to have seen me approximately eight to ten days after discharge but the unfortunate course of events negated this."

Augusta State Hospital superintendent Dr. John Patterson, said that all the usual procedures were followed in the case. He said that the law required no periodic check of her condition and the court made no such stipulation when it agreed to Mrs. Fisher's discharge. When asked if he would have released her he had no comment.

Dr. Patterson affirmed that the hospital had very little contact with her after her release and it had been almost a year and a half since anybody connected with the hospital had seen her.

In fact, hospital officials were not even aware that she had begun to have the old symptoms resurface and that she was receiving treatment from Dr. Kirkpatrick.

Absent from the public debate was Dr. Francis Sleeper who had retired from the Augusta State Hospital in 1963. Unfortunately, the recurrent tragedy was a blemish on a outstanding career; nonetheless, a large one.

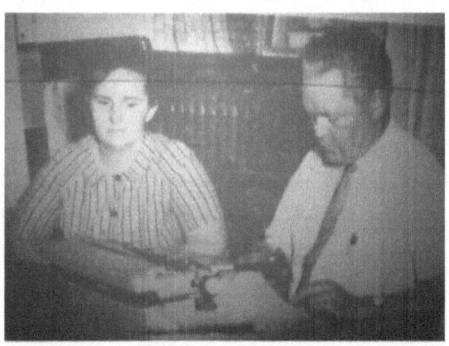

Court official takes a statement from Mrs. Fisher.

On July 1, 1966, Constance Fisher appeared before Kennebec County district court judge Roland J. Poulin, to be charged with three counts of murder, the same court at which she had appeared 12 years before for the identical offence.

She appeared pale and weary as she listened to Judge Poulin explain her rights. She was fitted with a yellow, blue and white cotton house dress, oxford shoes and white socks. She sat through the procedure with little emotion, sometimes stroking her tangled brown hair.

She kept her head bowed through most of the proceedings and her eyes closed. When asked to speak, her voice rose only slightly above a whisper. She sat alone this time, bereft of family and friends. Carl was not at the arraignment. He was excused from the hearing by Judge Poulin, who said he was in seclusion and under sedation.

As Constance Fisher stepped to the bar to confront the accusations against her, Judge Poulin asked her if she had the means to hire council and she said no. She then elaborated, " I have no money and I own nothing. My husband has a car but it belongs to his mother."

When asked if she wanted a court-appointed lawyer she answered, "It doesn't make any difference." Later, a court- appointed lawyer, George W. Perkins, a former district court judge, was tapped to defend her. She was then taken to the Kennebec County Jail and held without bail until the arraignment was completed the next week.

The arraignment was concluded on Tuesday, July 5. Mrs. Fisher sobbed loudly as Captain Drost recounted her explanation of the murders at the close of the hearing. It was the only evidence the judge needed to bind her over to the next session of Somerset County Superior Court. She entered no plea, but her defense argued, and was granted, that she be sent to the Augusta State Hospital for evaluation.

She was once again admitted to Middle Stone Female, a place for non-violent females, and placed on a suicide watch.

Ward notes describe her as being quiet and cooperative, sleeping much of the day. She was allowed to view television with other patients in the day room, one of the few escapes from the reality of her predicament. At least until the evening news came on.

The ward notes from July 7, 1966 read:

> *...After listening to tv, heard news about herself being at the state hospital. Came to the office door and said, "I think I need some medications." Was given Thorazine at 6:30 PM and 9:20 PM.*

From the start, it became apparent to Constance Fisher that things at the hospital would be different this time around.

Although the hospital staff was professional and her family still supportive, the second tragedy had all but extinguished the grace and mercy she had received for the first tragedy.

And there was no possibility of going home. Public sentiment would take care of that. Administrators and politicians whose careers were already on the line would take care of that. And with an enraged and befuddled public, perhaps it was safest for Mrs. Fisher to stay at the hospital.

And she wasn't going to jail either.

Perhaps it was punishment enough that Mrs. Fisher would realize the magnitude of her crimes on each occurrence of her children's birthdays, and death days. And the Mothers Day celebrations held at the hospital would be particularly cruel.

Ward notes from July 6, 1966 read:

> *She was found sobbing, lying on her bed. Asked if she would like a cold cloth for her head stated, " It could never help." My heart is broken, my home is empty. Why didn't I die....?*

And what of poor Carl whom she left to suffer in his own private hell? He would move towards the life of a complete recluse, and increasingly find his solace in a six-pack of beer.

On July 8, Constance penned a letter to Carl stating that she was sorry for what she had done, and said that if she could have held off another day or two the depression would have lifted and the incidents would not have happened.

She told Carl that she still loved him but would not blame him if he never wanted to see her again, and that she hoped he would not have a nervous breakdown over what she did.

In the ward notes for July 9, Mrs. Fisher made the following admission of guilt to a hospital attendant:

> *She started crying, asking for her children. Asked by attendant if she knew where her children were she said she did. Talked freely about the incident. Stated she drowned the boy first, then the big girl and finally the baby.*
> *Stated they struggled a little. Stated it happened between 10:00-10:30 am. Asked why she did it and stated she just had to. She had no one to take care of them and was so discouraged and depressed because she wasn't getting any better. Her medication*

was costing so much, their bills were pilling up. Her husband had to work and she kept getting worse.

...Told me that she hasn't heard any voices since she has been back this time, ... She told me she didn't want any more children because she is afraid the voices will come back. Stated that it's an awful experience to be depressed and hear voices.

In late July of 1966, Constance was given a battery of psychological evaluations that measured her intelligence, and emotional intelligence. The report read similar to those conducted in the 1954, having her "functioning in the superior range of intelligence."

... Her general level of judgment and comprehension and her ability to reason and think logically were lower but not deviant. In general she appears to be in relatively good contact with her environment at this point although she still is suffering from delusions of worthlessness and hopelessness which are rather realistic.

Mrs. Fisher is now quite concerned with death and hopelessness and had indicated that she still feels rather suicidal. She feels that people should not blame her for her deeds because she was unable to control herself. She is still concerned about not being in her right mind and feels quite lost because of this condition. The clinical picture is that of a psychotic depressive reaction. She is still suicidal and may attempt to commit suicide in the future.

On January 19, 1967, Constance Fisher was once again brought before a superior court to answer to the charge of murder. She appeared dressed in a dark gray plaid dress surrounded by three attendants. Seated within eyeshot was Carl, who stayed with her throughout the trial. She was counseled by her defense attorney George Perkins to plead innocent by reason of insanity.

The two-day trial consisted of crime scene evidence, a suicide note, and Mrs. Fisher's confession before Captain Albert Drost on the night of the murders. All of the evidence pointed in her direction.

Through the proceedings she sat motionless, although sometimes would make eye contact with Carl and nervously twist her handkerchief.

At 2 p.m. on January 19th, the state opened its argument against Mrs. Fisher, given by Assistant Attorney General Richard Cohen.

"We are here today for the purpose of trying, and yourselves are the finders of fact- three indictments of the State of Maine against Constance Margaret Fisher," Cohen said.

"The State will introduce evidence tying in the defendant with the events at Fairfield on June 30. The state will show that the defendant is indeed the perpetrator of these acts."

Cohen called seven witnesses to the stand, including Frederick Gould, Fairfield's chief of police, and Irving Goodof, a pathologist who showed that the children died of asphyxiation due to drowning.

Chief Gould was questioned about the "Dear Carl" note, written on the back of a greeting card, in which Mrs. Fisher confessed to the crime and sought her husband's forgiveness. Nurse Lydia Drummond was called as a witness to Mrs. Fishers confession before officer Drost.

Testimony described the Fishers' second try at a family, which started with Kathleen, born 11 months after Mrs. Fisher left the hospital. Kathleen was followed by Michael Jon, and then Natalie Rose. The first two births produced no post-partum reaction.

To those on the outside, everything seemed to be progressing smoothly and the Fisher couple, although without many close friends were slowly being assimilated into the community.

Constance Fisher gave all indications of continuing well on the road to recovery. There were no signs of abuse or neglect with the children, or any problems between her and Carl.

But there were signs to those close to Mrs. Fisher that shortly after the birth of her last child, she appeared to be slipping back into the illness that she had 12 years before.

The defense called only one witness, Dr. Walter Rohm, who had been observing Mrs. Fisher since her return to the Augusta State Hospital on July 6, 1966, and she was presently under his care. He was questioned under oath by Perkins:

Perkins:	*Did you reach any conclusions as to the mental condition of Mrs. Fisher?*
Dr. Rohm:	*Yes, she was and had been suffering from a mental disease at the time she entered the hospital and at the time the alleged crimes were committed.*
Perkins:	*Do you have an opinion as to her mental condition on June 30?*

Dr. Rohm:	*Yes, that she was suffering from a mental illness defined as Onirophonia. Its manifestation is a dream-like state of mind which normal people might experience as a nightmare. But for this person, Mrs. Fisher, this nightmare is real, a compelling reality. She has displayed a feeling of hopelessness, despair and pessimism.*
Perkins:	*Was Mrs. Fisher's conduct on June 30 consistent with you diagnosis?*
Dr. Rohm:	*Yes, it was.*

A closing summary was given by Cohen who then turned to the jurors and said:

> *I do not believe there can be any reasonable doubt from the evidence introduced in this trial, ladies and gentleman, evidence which I have just allowed you to hear, that it would be and is a fair and reasonable deduction for you to conclude from this evidence that the defendant, Mrs. Margaret Fisher was in fact the perpetrator of the acts alleged in these indictments, charging her with the crime of murder.*
>
> *Also, I know there is no question in any of our minds, that the deaths here in question are of a most tragic circumstance. Alluding to the psychiatric testimony, you heard the doctor testify that the defendant is suffering from a mental disease known as Onirophonia.*
>
> *You also heard testimony that after observations and examination a medical determination was made that the acts alleged by the state were a product of a mental disease, as will be well explained to you by the court when you are instructed on the appliance law...*
>
> *In closing I can only say, ladies and gentleman, that if after a careful consideration by you of all the evidence presented in this case you feel the alleged acts here involved were the product of a mental disease as defined to you by this court, the State would feel that this would certainly be a legitimate and rational conclusion to be drawn by you and I could have no quarrel with it.*

The fate of Constance Fisher was now in the hands of the jury. They were presented three options: innocent, guilty, or innocent by reason of insanity. The jury took 40 minutes of deliberation before returning with a unanimous verdict at 5:06 p.m.: Innocent by reason of insanity.

Constance Fisher sat motionless at the verdict. To her, capitol punishment might have been preferable to incarceration at the hospital, or the torture she felt in her own mind.

Life could provide her with nothing but remorse, knowing she had been given a second chance but somehow, some way, had let it slip from her.

On January 20, 1966, Constance Fisher was returned to the Augusta State Hospital where she was committed to the custody of the Commissioner of Mental Health and Corrections. The outlook for the rest of her life looked as cold and chilling as the bleak winter's day.

Φ Φ Φ Φ Φ Φ Φ Φ Φ Φ Φ Φ Φ Φ Φ Φ Φ Φ

CONSTANCE FISHER IS NOW 38 years old. She looks old and tired, her youthful beauty has all but disappeared.

She weighs close to 200 pounds. Her hair is graying, her countenance shows the years of struggle with an illness that has defied doctors and led to the death of her six children. She stares blankly at the TV sometimes, and carries on conversations with an unseen guest.

Her usual vivaciousness and zest for reading and learning are all but extinguished. The joys of parenting, watching the kids grow up and sharing their triumphs and tragedies, are a mocking illusion. Her crushed dreams of spending the golden years with Carl, with the children there to watch over them, enact a total eclipse of her heart

Visits by her in-laws, and friends are less and less frequent. Letters and inquiries of her well being are starting to tail off. As he had throughout, Carl Fisher remains a regular visitor, but even his visits bring little consolation.

An appraisal of Mrs. Fishers condition done on April 18, 1967, sums up her last stay at the hospital.

Patient's condition remains essentially unchanged over the third month of her present hospitalization. She remains quite inactive

around the ward, watching television most of the time or engaging in some small talk of trivialities with other patients. Patient was transferred today to Upper Marquardt South for further care.

She is unable to make friends with other patients in the admission service. This is most likely the result of the more chronic patients immediately telling new patients that the patient was involved in an act that they find repulsive. Steps have been made certain that patient would not easily be able to abscond.

With no goal for release, no carrot to chase, Constance Fisher's time at the hospital is spent in survival mode, with sleep, entertainments, and books her only escapes.

For Constance Fisher, the months turned into years with little change, with little hope, even when she is not beset by depression and suicidal thoughts. Her only consolation is that she has the final say if things get too bad. Dr. Sleeper called it "the quick exit into eternity."

A year-end summary from January 19, 1969 read:

There has been little, if any change in patient's condition during the last year. She mumbles to herself, apparently responding to auditory hallucinations. She is cooperative with the nursing staff but does not mingle with the other patients, preferring to remain alone. She is neat and tidy in her personal appearance and does ward chores as assigned.

The doctor's notes and summations read almost identical year after year.

Surprisingly, in January of 1972, Mrs. Fisher made another appeal to be released from the hospital. In a handwritten note she asked Dr. Abraham to consider her release.

Dear Dr. Abraham,

Do you think there is any chance that I can get out of here?
I think the next term of court is this month-so please let me know as soon as you can.
I am feeling very good, no mental aberrations of any kind. Hoping to hear from you soon.

Constance Fisher

The answer came later that month:

> *Mrs. Fisher has been doing well in Team 111 of the Ken-Som unit. There is, however, very little to add to her report of January 1972. She continues to work in the Message Service, but there is no vitality in her. She is aloof, withdrawn and delusional.*
>
> *It is the combined opinion of the treatment team and of myself that Mrs. Constance Fisher retains dangerous delusions regarding young children and therefore, she should not be discharged from this hospital.*

The three-paragraph summary read like a death sentence to Constance. Like a prisoner with no hope of parole, or pardon, she knew that life at the Augusta Mental Health Institute would be her lot until she breathed her last.

In August of 1973, a memo was issued by Dr. Abraham to Superintendent Roy Ettlinger who had only recently taken over as head of the hospital. It gave Ettlinger a synopsis of her history and her medical status. It would later provide Constance Fisher the opportunity to exit her troubles.

> *Mr. Ettlinger,*
>
> *Mrs. Fisher was admitted March 9, 1954 after having been accused of murdering her children. This was a Superior Court Commitment. An extensive examination on admission revealed no significant physical findings. Psychiatric examination revealed a psychotic process and she was diagnosed as suffering from Schizophrenia, paranoid type.*
>
> *Over the next five years, she improved sufficiently to warrant a request for a discharge and this was granted by order of Superior Court on May 6, 1959. She was readmitted on July 6, 1966 after the murder of another three children.*
>
> *Since then, Mrs. Fisher has remained confined in this hospital. She has continued withdrawn, busying herself with quiet activities such as sewing or knitting. She has no friends in this hospital. Her mood is one of resignation with occasional depression.*
>
> *Patient is still menstruating, but her husband was talked to by the treatment team and he stated that he would never take*

223

Connie home even for even a week-end. He made it clear to the treatment team and his wife that there would never be any sexual relations ever again between the two of them for fear that another child might be conceived.

He explained this to his wife and she accepted this decision. He made it clear to the team and his wife that there would not be any sexual relations between them.

It is possible that she will remain here for a long time yet. The prospect is bleak and we feel that a partial release would allow us to take her out on supervised activities.

One of her few visitors was Louise Bowker. She remained a friend and confidant to her sister, as would other family members. She saw yet another tragedy coming, but like a speeding train out of control, was helpless to stop it.

Louise would meet her sister in the day room, in the public area outside of the ward where her room was. The noise alone, she said, was enough to make a sane person crazy.

Usually upbeat at her visits, Constance was now talking more about wanting to die. She had no hope of going home, even if by some miracle the doctors and the court agreed that she could. A painful decision made by her husband guaranteed there would not be a second chance.

After 27 years of "for better or for worse", Carl Fisher informed her doctors that he had finally come to the end of his emotional resources. He would not seek a divorce or an annulment and would continue to support her materially. But the visits were over, and he would not take her back home under any circumstances.

March 17, 1973 was Carl's last recorded visit. It is not known what went or what was said as they met in the back of the crowded day room that overlooked the Kennebec River, so prominent now as it was approaching early spring flood stage.

To Constance, Carl's admission probably came as no surprise. For Carl, it was time to think about a future on his own.

It was recommended by hospital staff that a boarding home might be an option for Constance, but she balked at the idea. It appeared that from June on she had just one goal in mind, and she would accomplish it one way or another.

She intimated to Louise that the thought of spending the rest of her life at the hospital was too much for her and that she was thinking of committing suicide.

Her plan was to drown herself in the Kennebec River; death by water, the same way her children had died.

In the spring and summer months of 1973, Constance turned more and more to her Catholic faith. Ward notes showed that she became more withdrawn, and was having religious delusions. Her countenance and behavior was like that of a prisoner on death row waiting for the consummation of sentence.

She began to gather a collection of religious paraphernalia; sets of rosary beads, holy water, and prayer books. She seemed engrossed in one book in particular, a book on the lives of the saints.

On Wednesday, October 1st, 1973, Constance Fisher joined them in death by escaping from the hospital and drowning herself in the Kennebec River.

Was October 1, the day that Constance Fisher had chosen to die, or was it a day in which she felt so despondent, so overwhelmed, that she summoned the little resolve left and ended her miserable existence?

October 1st on the Catholic calendar, is a day of remembrance for the life of St. Therese, patron of the florist and the sick. She was called "Little Flower" for her love of children.

St. Therese had endured the death of four siblings, had a mentally ill father, and later contracted tuberculosis. She died of asphyxiation from water in her lungs.

Was Constance's death on this date by coincidence or was it her plan?

One thing was for sure- Constance Fisher's arduous battle with life was finally over.

* CHAPTER FOURTEEN *

RIVER RIDE

*"The Kennebec River borders the west side (of the hospital).
Its dark, cold flowing waters the boundary that separates
the privileged from the patients, would sometimes end
the lives of those trying to bridge the gulf."*

Alice Frost, 1937

Monday, October 1, 1973

CONSTANCE FISHER'S LAST DAY on earth was lived in the same drama she had lived out most of her life.

It was a chilly autumn day, with leaves showing bright colors in their transition from life to death. Constance awakened in her single room in south Stone, an open ward with a window view of the Kennebec River.

The temperature upon her arising was close to freezing, although by 2 p.m. it would reach a balmy 65 degrees. She dressed warmly in a blue cotton dress, clean and comely as usual.

After finishing breakfast around 7 a.m., Constance returned to her room and rested before undertaking her duties of dispensing mail to other patients in the messenger service she helped to run.

She had been noted at breakfast as appearing depressed and listless by a nurse on duty, but that was nothing new.

Around 8 a.m. Mrs. Fisher was questioned about her emotional state by Kenneth Thompson, a psychiatric aide who had noted her dreary disposition and haltering step. She was brought back into a secured area on the wing and interviewed by the resident RN, Mrs. Dugan. She was then seen briefly by Dr. Gerald Abraham at about 11 a.m., and he gave her something to take the edge off her anxiety.

Observation notes dated October 1, 1973 read:

> *"Connie was very depressed and hallucinating. Was brought to section 3 and interviewed by Dr. Abraham. Medication increased."*

Constance promptly slept through dinner and was not seen again until she was awakened at 2:30 p.m. by nurse Dugan.

She was not seen or heard from for the remainder of the afternoon. At the evening meal, which started at 5:00 p.m., her seat was empty. Her few friends said they had no knowledge of her whereabouts. After a three hour search of the wards, the grounds, and the out buildings, officials notified the state police that Mrs. Fisher was missing.

Hospital superintendent Roy Ettlinger then released a statement to the media:

> *"While there is concern on the part of the staff that she might be dangerous to herself, she is not considered to be dangerous to others. Mrs. Fisher is considered to have eloped and state and local police have begun a search for her."*

The incident made the front page of the next day's Waterville Morning Sentinel. A recount of the tragic incidents that had landed her in the hospital was given. Ettlinger was grilled as to how Mrs. Fisher could have slipped through the cracks.

Ettlinger said that Mrs. Fisher had grounds privileges at the institution but she did not have permission to leave the grounds. He later clarified that Mrs. Fisher was on a partial release by order of the Superior Court and had therefore been given the opportunity to leave the building, but only under staff supervision.

The furor over Mrs. Fisher's escape raged in the community. The Kennebec River was dragged but failed to produced a body. Local communities were scoured by state and local police departments. A rumor persisted that Mrs. Fisher had jumped to her death off the Memorial Bridge that spans the east and west sides of Augusta.

The fear of a mental patient with homicidal tendencies at large in the community fanned a fire across the city of Augusta and it's environs.

But 35 miles south, in the neighborhood of the former Fisher home in Fairfield Center, a sighting of Mrs. Fisher had been reported. At approximately 8 p.m. Constance Fisher was said to have knocked on the door of the residence of Gerald and Gabrielle Raymond, who lived just across the field from the former Fisher home.

"She came pounding at the door and my wife told her to get the hell out," said, Gerald Raymond. "A few days later we read in the paper that she had drowned in the river."

Questions about Constance Fisher's whereabouts, and how she managed to escape, now loomed as large as the dilemma that caused her incarceration in the first place.

Concern amongst her family was also at code red. "The whole week of her being missing was cold and rainy," Louise Bowker recalled.

"We were hoping and praying that she was all right, that she had found refuge somewhere and was safe from the cold."

The speculation ended peacefully on Saturday morning October 6, about 10:30 am.

It was the first day of hunting season and an unidentified man and his son out duck hunting discovered the bloated body of Mrs. Fisher.

It had been caught up in the reeds and washed up along the west bank of the Kennebec River in South Gardiner. Her fully clothed body was found with several strands of rosary beads around her neck, and wearing the same dress she was last seen in at the hospital.

Louise Bowker recalled getting the phone call from police that Constance had been found.

"When we found out she was dead, it was a consolation to know that she would not have to suffer anymore. It is like a person with cancer who dies, you miss them but you are glad they are out of their pain."

The Gardiner police exhumed the body from its water grave and delivered it to the morgue at the Gardiner branch of the Maine Medical Center. It was then examined by Dr. Henry Ryan, who estimated that the body had been in the water for several days. He issued a death certificate that read:

> Name: Constance M Fisher.
> Occupation: Housewife.
> Age: 44
> Mother: Unknown
> Father: Unknown
> Social Security #: Unknown
> Death was caused by: Asphysixia, Drowning. Suicide.

As with the death of her children, Constance Fisher had met her end by water.

On October 8, 1973, a service was held for Constance Fisher at the Gallant Funeral Home in Waterville, and later at St. Bridget's church in North Vassalboro, where Carl Fisher was now a member.

Her remains were then taken to the Saint Francis Catholic Cemetery in Waterville where she was interred with her six children. To her side was left a spot for Carl, who would join the family reunion 17 years later.

Φ Φ Φ Φ Φ Φ Φ Φ Φ Φ Φ Φ Φ Φ Φ Φ Φ Φ

D R. JACOBSOHN WAS ON staff at the Augusta State Hospital when Mrs. Fisher escaped and committed suicide, an act that became a controversy and the probe of an investigation done by State Senator Walter Hichens.

He said that her suicide was not due to a lack of proper treatment or lack of responsible supervision but rather a resignation to the fact that she would rather die than spend the rest of her life as a prisoner/patient at the hospital.

"When her release was judged to be impossible and that she had no future outside of the hospital whatsoever, because of that realization, she committed suicide," Dr. Jacobsohn said.

According to the most popular report, Mrs. Fisher had escaped the

AMHI grounds, walked towards the downtown section of Augusta and jumped off the south side of the Memorial Bridge and into the Kennebec River. Dr. Jacobsohn was quick to dispel that theory as false.

"Mrs. Fisher did not jump off the bridge but had walked down to the river side that bordered the property and cast herself fully clothed into the river," he said.

At the heart of the controversy was a grounds pass issued to Mrs. Fisher that allowed her to move freely around the hospital grounds, even to the river front which was the complex's west boundary.

Dr. Jacobsohn said that she had earned the privilege of having a grounds pass and that doctors felt it might add some dressing to a very bland life.

He was aware of the fact that the river might present an appealing option in the event she determined to commit suicide.

"With grounds privileges there was nothing to stop her from going into the river if that was the method she chose to end her life."

Senator Hichens, chairman of the health institutional services committee, blamed her disappearance and death on what he called the "irresponsible pass system" used by the hospital. It seemed that even in death the system had let Constance Fisher down.

Hitchens placed the blame for the drowning on three state officials, William Kearns, mental health and corrections commissioner, Dr. William Schumacher, mental health director, and Ettlinger. He told the media that Constance Fisher would still be alive if they had heeded his warning.

He had warned state officials on several occasions that patients like Mrs. Fisher should not be given passes either on or off hospital grounds.

"We mentioned Mrs. Fisher in particular and Dr. Schumacher replied that she was no risk on a pass privilege," Hichens said. "If she did any damage, he said it would be to herself." When I asked if that was something to worry about, he said it was not really a concern."

Two years earlier, after violations had occurred at both the Augusta and Bangor Mental Health hospitals, Hichens had suggested the that pass system be discontinued until it could be reevaluated and tweaked.

Ettlinger followed that increased suicide risks are inherent in the active treatment program in which Mrs. Fisher and others had been involved.

Hichens was also opposed to the shift in treatment mode for patients which was calling for less time in the state hospitals and an earlier transition into the community. He cited several cases when patients were released prematurely from the Augusta State Hospital, and the results were disastrous.

"There was a man in Eliot whose wife and mother were patients at Augusta," Hichens explained. "They were both discharged, and within six months after they left the hospital they were both dead."

"There were others who called to tell me that their relatives had been sent off to boarding homes and they had received no notification that these relatives were going to be moved. The hospital just pushes them out, whether they can take it or not."

Hichens went on to point out that Ettlinger was not even a psychologist or a psychiatrist, the first superintendent in the hospital's history not to be so trained.

It seemed that Ettlinger had been given a mandate to shrink the hospital's size and its budget. He succeeded in the former, but when re-admittance rates skyrocketed, the hospital's financial resources went into depression.

Although not agreeing entirely with his approach, the Kennebec Journal took sides with Hichens on the issue.

In an editorial they wrote:

> ...*The pass system at the state hospitals, also the work of imperfect humans, may have failed too... In some mental illness the patient must be protected from himself. In the most recent Augusta situation, reports that the patient was missing were soon followed by the note that the patient should be considered dangerous only to herself. A few days later her body was recovered from the Kennebec River. In dismal fashion, the diagnosis seemed confirmed. (1)*

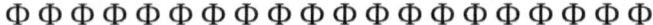

232

I WAS ONCE AGAIN JOINED by Michael Shepherd as we tried to reenact the last steps of Constance Fisher.

As we drove into the complex of the former Augusta State Hospital, I was struck by the enormity of the complex and the noble purpose for which it was conceived.

I could not help but think of Dr. Isaac Ray as I looked up three stories to the portion of the Stone Building where he lived and re-wrote one of the most famous works in the history of forensic psychiatry.

What would Dr. Ray think today of the total retreat from moral treatment for the unfulfilled promise of anti-psychotic drugs?

What would Dr. Ray think about the buildings that once housed the many patients in need of the hospital's services, now being occupied by state employees?

Perhaps he might want to fire off one of the cannons just beneath us at the old military arsenal, pointing it directly at the chamber of the legislature.

It was easy to let my mind wander back to the case of Moses Butterfield. Butterfield lived in the Stone Building for the last 25 years of his life, never learning the why of his actions, left only with the haunting memory that his hand had put to death the people he had loved most in life.

I climbed the large granite steps to the entry of the Stone Building as Michael looked on.

How many grieving, shipwrecked lives had climbed those steps over the past century and a half? If those stones could cry out what stories they would tell!

A great dichotomy, I supposed. Human kind at its lowest being treated by human kind at its best. I was reminded of the story of an American journalist in China during World War 11 who watched a Sister of Mercy cleaning the gangrenous sores of wounded soldiers.

"I wouldn't do that for a million dollars!" the journalist remarked. The sister, without pausing from her work, replied, "Neither would I."

I peered in to the waiting area that had received a disheveled Constance Fisher on two occasions, and looked over at the stairs she must have exited in incredible joy when she was released from the hospital in 1959.

I thought of the thousands who had entered through that front door, many against their will; not because it was a bad place but because it was a new place and they feared the unknowns that might be hidden beyond the door.

For others, the hospital must have granted a blessed freedom from the stresses that agitated their illness. And it gave others a hope that somebody in there might have an answer to the problems that were decimating their lives.

Walking back to my car I viewed a panorama of decaying buildings, overgrown brush, and unkempt lawns. I noticed that portions of the property were up for sale.

Once a hub of activity the complex was now silent. Once a small city and community where the drama of life played out, was now virtually void of human presence. Much of the grounds, once so immaculately landscaped in accordance to the Kirkbride plan, was now a series of asphalt parking lots.

The site had lost its purpose and function in my generation, much to the grief of its founders, I was sure.

Michael interrupted my musings by saying he thought he had a plausible route for Mrs. Fishers escape and descent into the river. We made our way down from the Stone Building, past the small gazebo and headed west towards a field and then a wooded area that separated the buildings from the river.

We followed the remnants of a path, covered mostly by overgrowth and underbrush. The path made its way down to the river front past the granite buildings that were once part of the U.S. military arsenal built in 1827 and later given to the hospital to be used for forensic patients.

We were both caught by the breathtaking view of a granite embankment with at least a 20 foot drop into the river. Given the fact that Mrs. Fisher was a heavy-set middle-aged woman with nothing to grab but a slippery stone wall, a plunge from here meant certain death into the moving river.

But there were no witnesses to the event and that is what made us re-evaluate our theory. The major problem with the arsenal route was that there would be plenty of witnesses. The three granite structures that surrounded the embankment would have been full of patients, and personnel conducting surveillance at the maximum security building.

We left the premise with little but conjecture. But on our way back to the car, I flagged a gentleman who appeared to be an employee at the Riverview facility next door.

He told us that he had been a longtime employee at the Augusta Mental Health Institute, and was familiar with the Fisher case.

Even though he did not work there at the time of Mrs. Fisher's suicide, Justin Pottle * had worked the route several times on other escapes and suicide attempts in the river. He offered this explanation:

"If she was coming out of the Stone Building, she probably headed towards the Gazebo, and went down into the fields," he said. "From there, she could find cover in the wooded area that leads down to the river."

He figured the length of the final walk to be about an eighth of a mile from the entrance of the Stone Building to the river bank. He agreed with Dr. Jacobsohn that Constance Fisher had not jumped off the Memorial Bridge but had carefully planned her route through the woods so as not to be seen.

There was something else that puzzled me. I told Michael that according to the police report, Mrs. Fisher's body had floated all the way to South Gardiner, a 7-mile journey by car from the hospital grounds.

There had been numerous suicides in the river from the hospital, and a number who had plunged to their deaths off the Memorial Bridge. But most of the bodies, if not all, were found in the general vicinity, occasionally making it down as far as nearby Hallowell or Farmingdale.

I sensed there might be something significant about Mrs. Fisher's unlikely journey to her final resting place.

The swift-moving river current heightened by the recent October rains, probably moved her body through the eddies that lined the east side of the river. Somehow, it managed to get through the log flumes that cross the river in Hallowell and again in Farmingdale, which in earlier times were used to catch stray timbers during log drives.

In Farmingdale, a large land mass divided the river into an east and west channel, but somehow the body did not drag ashore there.

Depending upon the tide, large sand bars would emerge from the river bed, sure to catch and hang up a drifting body at some point during the day or night. And as it entered Gardiner, the body would have to contend with the concrete piers that support the bridge from Gardiner to Randolph.

Having made it this far, the body would have had clear sailing all the way to Merrymeeting Bay where it would encounter the sharp currents and whirlpools known as "Hells Gates" before heading out to sea.

But Mrs. Fishers body came to rest on the west shore of the river, in a wooded area in South Gardiner, almost at the foot of Mount Tom.

Was it possible for something as large as a 200-pound object to cross the river and to make it all the way from Augusta to Mount Tom? My limited experience on the river told me no.

Not wanting to rely solely upon my own judgment, I sought the help of a friend, Mike Costigan who owned a home on the river, just up from where Mrs. Fishers body was recovered. He told me he would be happy to take me by boat the probable path the body had traveled.

On September 22, taking advantage of superb weather, we boarded his 22-ft run-about and made our way down to the arsenal where I concluded that Mrs. Fisher first entered the Kennebec River.

Mike had been navigating that corridor of the river for almost 20 years, but still used the utmost caution in avoiding the different barriers, rocks, and man made obstacles. We passed under the Memorial Bridge, turned, and began to retrace her journey to South Gardiner.

As we finished the 6.5 nautical mile journey, I had some questions for Mike.

"What are the chances that a body, or even a small raft, could make the journey from Augusta all the way to South Gardiner without running ashore, getting caught in a log flume, or hanging up on a sand bar?"

His slowness in response told me he had much to consider.

"Okay, how about running aground on either of the islands, or the exposed rocks at low tide, or maybe even the piers holding the Gardiner Bridge?"

Mike paused again before answering. "Even with all the right conditions, wind, tides, current, I would say slim to none."

Mike then drove to the location where Mrs. Fisher's body had been found, most likely unchanged even after 38 years. It was on the west shore of the river, and not in an area influenced by current or eddies. It seemed like an odd place for the body to have ground ashore.

As I looked up I could plainly see the grounds of the Oakland estate, built in the 1830's for Robert Hallowell Gardiner, one of the wealthiest and most influential citizens in the state. The property was later occupied by a former Maine Governor, William Tudor Gardiner.

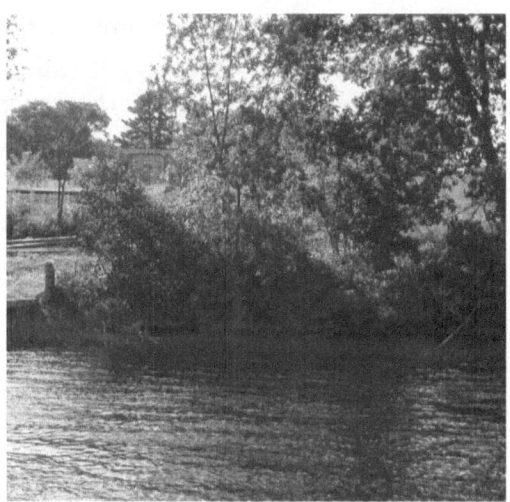

Location where the body of Constance Fisher was found by hunters. In the background is the mansion once owned by former Maine governor William Tudor Gardiner.

Born into wealth and influence, Governor Gardiner was a deeply religious man and one of the leading Episcopal layman in the state. He attended Harvard University, graduating in 1914 before enlisting in the Army and fighting in the European theatre of the war.

The war greatly impacted Gardiner, and he now saw politics, not warfare, as the best way to exact change.

Gardiner was elected to several terms in the Maine House of Representatives and in 1928 was nominated as the Republican candidate for governor. Gardiner was elected as governor of Maine for two terms, serving from 1928-1932.

In Governor Gardiner's inaugural address, he noted Mainers left indigent by accident or illness, should be the entire state's responsibility.

He explained that the well being of all Maine citizens should be the highest priority, even over the needs of commerce and industry.

Although Governor Gardiner had to deal with an unprecedented lack of finances, as his term ran through the beginning years of the Great Depression, he remained true to this ideal.

After squeezing as much money out of the legislature as he could to help run the mental health hospitals in Augusta and Bangor, he petitioned the private sector for monies to enable their continued operation.

Where Dorothea Dix had failed in her attempt to secure endowment for the hospital at the federal level, Gardiner did at the state. He pushed a bill through the legislature to secure that trust monies established for these institutions could not be spent anywhere else.

To the Augusta State Hospital he guaranteed bequests totaling almost $ 60,000 would remain in perpetuity to service the needs of those at the hospital. A similar endowment was made to the psychiatric hospital in Bangor.

It was also under Gardiner's leadership that the Department of Health and Welfare was established with the mental hospitals and the Pineland school for the mentally retarded chief among it's concerns.

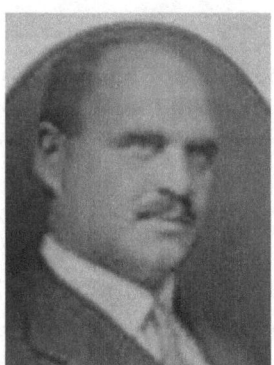

William Tudor Gardiner, c. 1929
It was Gardiner's ambition that life, liberty and the pursuit of happiness
be made available to all citizens of the state. He had a particular
concern for the plight of the mentally ill and handicapped.

As I looked up from the weeded area where Mrs. Fisher's body had been found and saw the Oakland mansion in full view, I had a startling but delightful thought.

Could it be that in one last fateful gesture, Constance Fisher made an appeal to the politicians of Maine not to forget those whose lives had been destroyed by the cruelness of mental illness? And to the rest of us that like it or not, we are still our brother's keeper.

* CHAPTER FIFTEEN *

CARNAGE

"She could have left me just one of them..."

Carl Fisher, June 30, 1966

UNFORTUNATELY, THE VICTIMS OF mental illness are not just the sufferers.

The Fisher children, the Butterfield children, the Bergen family were all victims as well. Innocent victims. And sometimes the worst pain is felt by the ones left standing, like Warren and Ursula Marcoux.

The tragedies, all three of them, left a black hole in their hearts and lives. In a little over a decade they had lost six grandchildren and watched the one they had raised since childhood repeatedly self-destruct.

Even a change of scenery, a move to Arizona, offered little more than an aspirin to ease their pain.

So many questions left unanswered. Had they not tried their hardest to rear their foster daughter right? Had they not given her every opportunity to succeed, including the expense of private schools?

Maybe they should not have sent her away to the convent school at such an early age. Maybe they could have been more supportive of her marriage and helped with the kids more. Maybe they could have been more proactive when she was sick... On and on the painful analysis goes. Maybe it wouldn't have made any difference anyway.

Warren Marcoux had felt that it was a mistake for Constance to move to Snow Pond shortly after she was married.

Too much isolation, too little human interaction. Being alone all day with the children was enough to drive anyone mad. Maybe he should have voiced his observation to Constance instead of just complaining about it to his wife.

And he could not understand why Constance had made a similar choice when she and Carl moved to Fairfield Center. Again, there was no phone, no lifeline for help, and it was too remote for people to observe if there was a need for outside intervention.

And Ursula, maybe she could have been a little more involved in helping Constance raise her children even though at the time, she still had small ones of her own.

But the Marcoux family would have pitched in in a heartbeat if they knew the extent of her suffering. They would have taken the kids and given her a respite. As with most breakdowns in human communication, nothing was said because of pride, guilt, or shame.

In retrospect, Louise Bowker said there were three things the family might have done differently in avoiding both tragedies: Insist that they had a telephone, helped out more with the children, and availed themselves of the services at the Augusta State Hospital.

To their credit, the family attempted to move on and shunned the opportunity to live in the "what ifs" of the past.

In the Constance Fisher tragedy however, there was none who suffered more than Carl.

Carl Fisher decided to stay with his wife after the first tragedy even though the Catholic Church surely would have granted him an annulment. And who would have blamed him if he decided that enough was too much, and left her to start a new life?

But Carl forgave and reconciled with his wife. He waited patiently while Constance received treatment, not knowing if she would ever be well enough to return to him.

And when his dreams did come true, they were only to be destroyed again by the return of Constance's illness. Yet even then he remained faithful to her, never blaming her directly for all the pain and sorrow. But it took it's toll on a tough, caring man.

In an evaluation done by Margaret Nelson at the Augusta State Hospital shortly after Constance was recommitted in 1966, Mrs. Nelson gave the following snapshot of a smoldering wick ready to go out:

> *The husband is a tall, graying, rather slender man with a prominent nose and a sad, shy manner. Tears came into his eyes, and he actually wept during the interview, but gradually became more composed and talked more easily.*

In the years that followed, there was much speculation about Carl Fisher.

Was he a saint? An enabler? Mentally ill himself? Much of the talk around Fairfield Center, both before and after the second murders, was questioning who in their right mind would put themselves in a position for the same tragedy to happen again.

Indeed, Mr. Fisher might have been an excellent candidate for analysis by his wife's physicians.

In Carl's defense, he was told plainly by doctors that his wife had recovered, and that having a new family would be therapy for her. And other than the two post partum aberrations, his wife had been sensible, responsible, a good mother and a good wife.

Carl Fisher was an enigma. Was his love for Constance so strong that he could withstand calamity that would send most men packing? Or was it that he had no backbone and was under the spell of a sociopathic wife? It was a question I posed to Dr. Jacobsohn.

"I am not surprised by his behavior and not surprised that most people would think otherwise," he said. "He took the role of a husband seriously. He had the mentality of 'taking a bullet for a friend,' and that is what he did for his wife. I see no illness or character defect there."

Dr. Jacobsohn felt he had a genuine devotion to his wife and she to him. "He took his marriage vows seriously. I can understand this. There are people in this world that take their commitments seriously."

Whatever the context of their relationship, their love for each other was undeniable. Constance wrote this poem to Carl while in the hospital the second time, in 1970:

Silvery willows by a moonlit pool, Breezes whispering--cool, cool, cool. And up yonder moonlit hill, I hear the call of whip-poorwill, whippoorwill, whippoorwill

And the moon and stars above All speak of love, love, love. O love of mine come here with me and sit beneath the willow tree To you my heart and the whippoorwill say, O sweetheart mine, please stay, stay, stay

O God above please bless me here and this love of mine I hold so dear. And through the years we will always remember This lovely scene and our love so tender. Whatever else the years may bring When I think of this moment, my heart will sing; Sing more than the breeze or the whippoorwill, Of this love we found neath a moonlit hill. A love so deep, a love so true, This deathless love that I have for you.

The time came however, when the burden of caring for Constance became too much. His visits became infrequent. He refused to take her off on restricted leave. And then, when Constance became delusional, and overcome by religious obsessions, he stopped seeing her completely.

He continued to support her financially, using some of the proceeds from the sale of his house and cabin on Snow Pond to pay for a private room.

Although Carl found some relief in pulling away from Constance, his world would be racked once again by Constance's suicide, wondering if his actions had helped precipitate it.

Paul Fisher, Carl's younger brother, said that Carl was stunned over the death of his wife.

"He was very upset over Constance's suicide. He moved back in with my mother for a while before moving to Vassalboro."

Paul Fisher said that Carl developed a neuro muscular disorder that gave him great pain with every movement. Despite this, he continued to work as a cook at the Maine Central Railroad until he retired in 1980, at age of 60.

Former neighbor, Don Wilson, said he had heard that Carl had taken up drinking again after his wife's suicide, to which he commented, "Under the circumstances, what man in his right mind wouldn't have?"

His last address was listed at Nowell Street in Winslow, Maine, where he was being taken care of in an assisted living arrangement.

Carl Merrill Fisher died on September 26, 1990 at the Maine Medical Center, Thayer Unit, the same hospital where his last three children were autopsied, the same institution where his wife was unsuccessfully treated.

His death report said the cause of death was cardio pulmonary failure. Or, in layman's terms, he died of a broken heart.

Another casualty of the tragedy was the priesthood of Father Joseph Brannigan.

Father Brannigan conducted the graveside burial of the last three Fisher children at St. Francis Catholic cemetery in Waterville. It was a sight he will never forget. He later commented on the scene,

"The three small caskets, the grief on Carl's face; the unanswered questions, it left a lasting impact."

After the funeral he stayed in touch with Mr. Fisher until Carl chose to end their friendship.

"I just can't see you anymore," he told Father Brannigan. "You remind me too much of what has happened."

Shortly after the tragedy, Brannigan left the priesthood and became a mental health clinician, helping to found a mental health clinic in southern Maine called Shalom House, where he served as its executive director.

Brannigan was also elected to the Maine House of Representatives and then to the Maine Senate where he has served as chairman for the Health and Human Services committee.

Senator Brannigan believes that there were several guilty parties in he Constance Fisher tragedy. He cites flaws in the mental health system, the lack of follow up on Mrs. Fisher, and even Carl Fisher.

"The second time was no surprise to Carl, he should have known better than to have allowed the same things to happen all over again."

Brannigan believes however, there was a silver lining in the dark cloud. He said the case brought a greater scrutiny on forensic cases, greater accountability within the mental health system, and a change in the statutes governing the committal and release of the mentally ill.

"The Fisher tragedy changed the laws, not only in the state of Maine but the whole nation," Brannigan said.

Perhaps the greatest loss in the tragedy is what might have become of the Fisher children.

They came from an excellent gene pool of attractive, intelligent, hard working people. They had a loving extended family of grandparents, aunts, uncles, and cousins as close-knit as you can get.

And the United States had entered into one of the most prosperous times in its history. The greatest generation had given birth to the most privileged generation, perhaps in the history of the world. As never before, there would be opportunities for education, employment, and living the American dream.

But for Richard, Daniel, Deborah, Kathleen, Michael Jon, and Natalie Rose Fisher, they would never have the chance to enjoy those opportunities. Never have the chance to fulfill their dreams.

CHAPTER SIXTEEN

MOVING FORWARD, STEPPING BACKWARD

"It is a fact too well known to need be elucidated, that the insane cannot be successfully treated with curative means at their homes, and among their friends, and that well regulated asylums alone afford the requisite facilities for restoring to health and reason the most unfortunate class of community."

Isaac Ray, 1842.

MEDICAL SCIENCE AND THE judicial system are in agreement on this one point: the mentally ill are not the enemy, their illness is.

And a heinous enemy it is; one that ruins lives, destroys families, and devours fortunes.

And the enemy is growing. The World Health Organization estimates that by 2020, mental illness will be the second leading cause of death and disability in the world.

There are now more suicides than homicides each year in America, and experts are saying that perhaps 90 % of the victims were suffering from treatable psychiatry disorders.

America is feeling an economic strain from the problem as well.

Over 5 million people in the United States suffer an acute episode of mental illness each year, with the price of the illness in hospitalization, treatment, and lost wages, in excess of $80 billion.

The sadness is that mental illness could be thwarted to a much greater degree if our national attitude and resources were marshaled against it.

As one writer said, "It is shocking but true that we know the atom today better than we know the mind that knows the atom."

That was written in 1940. But instead, our national commitment has been in developing weapons of mass destruction, rather than fighting diseases that destroy.

And the medical community continues it's unfruitful path of looking for a quick fix to an inconvenient truth. The truth that far too many of the chronically mentally ill are treated with a check, and prescription, then thrust out into communities that neither want them or are able to care for them.

What has become obvious is that the elimination, or even the control of mental illness, has proved far more difficult than merely swallowing a pill. The human psyche in all of its complexities must be treated on many fronts, just as the original architects of moral treatment tried to tell us.

In what has become a national disgrace, many of our country's mentally ill wander the streets in an aimless stab at life, targets for gangs and thieves. They fill the homeless shelters, soup kitchens, and emergency rooms. They end up in jails and prisons for crimes they are not responsible for committing. It is déjà vu all over again. It is back to pre-1840 conditions in America.

There was a time in our nations recent history when this travesty of American life was not swept under the carpet.

Newly elected president John F. Kennedy was a champion for the cause of the mentally ill, inspired mainly because it had struck a family member. His sister, Rosemary, suffered from mental disease that was accentuated by a lack of proper treatment.

Kennedy sought to enact mental health legislation that would stress prevention, care, and place treatment facilities in every community.

In 1963, he led Congress in passing the Community Mental Health Care Act. The legislation was ground breaking. For the first time in 109 years the federal government was going to get directly involved in the health care system.

Kennedy outlined his plan in the following speech given in the spring of 1963:

> *I have sent to the congress today a series of proposals to fight mental illness and mental retardation. These two afflictions have been long neglected. They occur more frequently, affect more people, require more prolonged treatment, cause more individual and family suffering than any other condition in American life.*
>
> *It has been tolerated too long. It has troubled our Nation's conscience, but only as a problem unpleasant to mention, easy to postpone and despairing of solution. The time has come for a great national effort. New medical and scientific and social tools and insights are now available....If we launch a brand new mental health program now, it will be possible within a decade or two to reduce the number of patients now under custodial care by 50% or more.*
>
> *Here more than in any other area, an ounce of prevention is worth more than a pound of cure. For prevention is far more desirable for all concerned. It is far more economical and it is far more like to be successful...*
>
> *We as a nation have neglected too long the mentally ill and the mentally retarded. It affects all of us and it affects us as a country. I am hopeful that beginning today this country will move with a great national effort in this field so vital to the welfare of our citizens.* (1)

Kennedy believed that by the 1970's, the entire country would be covered by in-between mental health centers. He envisioned 2,000 community mental health centers that would dispense drugs, monitor progress, and ease patients back into society... when they were ready to return.

The larger state-run hospitals, though scaled down, would serve as a safety net and a refuge for those with chronic conditions.

Unfortunately, the legislation would never be fully implemented. The president's untimely death played a part in it, as did the civil rights movement, and the Vietnam War.

And the "wonder drugs" said to arrive to the rescue, did not live up to the pharmaceutical companies boasts.

Regrettably, Americans instead became pre-occupied with another Kennedy vision; landing a man on the moon.

Without Kennedy's passion and leadership, mental health reform and legislation took another course. It took on a new name and adapted new core values. The new movement became known as Deinstituionalization.

Sociologists have called Deinstitutionalization one of the greatest social experiments of the 20th century. It has also became one of the greatest medical controversies.

In theory, the tenets of Deinstituionalization are noble and its ends desirable. Quick stays at the hospital instead of patients becoming institutionalized... A timely transfer from the hospital to a halfway house... Recovering patients slowly assimilated back into the community...

And patients would have the right to choose their treatment options and would no longer feel, and in some cases be, "committed" to an institution.

The advent of revolutionary new drugs to cure or at least curb symptoms would make it all possible. The day of the large, state-run, "everything under one roof" hospital was going be a thing of the past.

In Deinstitutionalization, the large institution was seen as part of the problem, not the solution.

And the savings incurred by closing these large white elephants, and selling off their prime land holdings, would more than pay for the new clinics and halfway houses being proposed. They might even pay for new research to help find the cause and cure for mental maladies.

In 1965, the Social Security Act shifted about 50 percent of mental health costs from the state to the federal government. The federal government now had the power to pull the plug on the large mental hospitals that they considered to be an overall drain on the economy.

Together with state legislatures, they decided the monies could be better spent elsewhere, although a portion of it would go directly to the mental health consumer.

They embraced Deinstitutionalization, not because it was proven to be a better therapeutic model, but because it would save money and silence the ever increasing patients rights advocates and their litigations.

In this they made a significant miscalculation. In 1969, the budget to run the new community mental health care initiative ran about 143 million. In 2011, the projected cost to taxpayers is a whopping 11 billion, an almost 8000 % increase.

The major costs increase has been caused by the revolving door syndrome of patients in constant demand of services, who, in need of triage, are only getting band aids.

In the early 1970's the Augusta State Hospital, then known as the Augusta Mental Health Institute, instituted a massive campaign to downsize its population, with the goal of closing its doors.

From 1971-1976 administrators succeeded in dropping the patient census from 1,500 to 350, and scaled down the professional staff. Ready or not, patients where released back in the communities. They crowded poorly staffed boarding homes and halfway houses, while others chose life on the streets.

While provision was made for patients to live independently, little was done to reduce the dysfunction that helped create their illness to begin with.

Then there was the problem of an increasing population of those in need of mental health services. In 1958, Constance Fisher's last full year at the hospital, the Augusta State Hospital housed 1,800 patients. The facility built to replace it, Riverview Psychiatric Center, contains 100 beds.

In 1958, the population of the state of Maine was roughly 750,000. In 2010, the population of the state of Maine was up to 1.25 million.

Question: Where are Maine's mentally ill now being treated, and how?

It would be interesting to know what Dr. Francis Sleeper would have thought of Deinstitutionalization. He never commented on it publicly. His son Frank, however, did in his book, "**Augusta**,"

He writes of the Augusta State Hospital:

> *This is one of the oldest hospitals for the mentally ill in the country. Its second superintendent was Isaac Ray, one of this country's most famous psychiatrists, who worked closely with Dorothea Dix, a native of Hamden, Maine, to bring the mentally ill out of jails.*

> *It's interesting to think about how Dr. Ray and Miss Dix*
> *would view the status of the mentally ill in much of this country*
> *now. In trying to place them back into the community, have we*
> *sentenced them to be homeless or put them back into jails?*
>
> *... Under the superintendence of Dr. Francis H. Sleeper,*
> *the institution reached its population peak in the late 1940's and*
> *early 1950's, and then fell as drugs to alleviate mental illness*
> *were discovered.*
>
> *But today, who or what insures that these suffering people*
> *will take their drugs once back in the community?*

On a winter night in 1996, the entire country would be reminded of just how great a price could be paid if they didn't.

On the evening of January 27, 1996, Mark Bechard a 38-year old Waterville, Maine, resident, walked three quarters of a mile through the rain from his apartment to the Servants of the Blessed Sacrament Convent.

Without warning he broke through the locked door of the rectory and made his way to the chapel where eight nuns had just finished their evening prayers.

Bechard encountered several of the nuns in the hallway, and in an animal-like frenzy, battered sisters Marie Julien Fortin, Edna Mary Cardozo and Mary Anna DiGiacomo with his fists untill they fell to the ground. He then stabbed them repeatedly with a kitchen knife.

His rampage extended into the chapel where another nun, Patricia Keane knelt in prayer. Bechard began to beat her with a cane which broke under the force of the blows. He then picked up a two-foot statue of the Virgin Mary and began bludgeoning the sister with it.

Officers responding to a 911 call burst into the sanctuary with guns raised to end the massacre. In the wake of the tragedy, there were two dead, Sisters Cardozo and Fortin. Sisters DiGiacomo and Keane, both brutally battered, suffered multiple wounds but survived.

Questions as to how the gentle, likeable, and talented young man could suddenly turn into a monster, were directed to the psychiatric community. Questions as to how the tragedy was allowed to happen in public, were directed towards state lawmakers.

Outrage over the tragedy was deafening and most of it aimed at the Department of Human Services for downsizing the Augusta Mental Health Institute before an alternative plan had been thoroughly tested.

Living alone and not taking his medicines in the weeks before the attack, Bechard was on a collision course with disaster. Neighbors reported hearing him screaming in the middle of the night, but could do nothing. Under state law Bechard could not be touched until something happened, or until it was too late.

It was the kind of tragedy that mental health workers and law enforcement agents had been warning authorities about. Workers knew that many of the patients being released were not only a danger to themselves but to others. And law enforcement officials knew they were helpless to intervene untill after the fact.

The dilemma remains unresolved. The proper balance between the safety of the community and the rights of those suffering from mental illness has yet to be struck.

The massacre turned the city of Waterville on its ear, the same way the Constance Fisher murders had decades earlier.

Mark Bechard and Constance Fisher had, in fact, much in common. Although separated by a generation, they grew up in the same city, attended the same church, and came from similar family backgrounds.

They were both described as intelligent, attractive, and congenial with apparently bright futures. They both saw their worlds destroyed by the ravages of an illness that caused the lives of others to be destroyed as well.

Both spent time at and ended up in the same mental hospital. And they both suffered the deadly consequences of the move to empty the Augusta State Hospital of its patients before they were ready to leave it.

Φ Φ Φ Φ Φ Φ Φ Φ Φ Φ Φ Φ Φ Φ Φ Φ Φ Φ

BY THE TURN OF the 21st century, national Deinstitutionalization had left a legacy of homelessness, crime, and patients in dire need of treatment, left to fend for themselves. Jails and prisons had now become the de-facto mental institutions, leaving social scientists to coin a new term: re-institutionalization.

An internet columnist made a succinct evaluation of the situation:

> *Jails have now become society's primary mental institutions, though few have the funding or expertise to carry out that role properly...*
>
> *The well intentioned Deinstitutionalization movement, which started with the noble aim of treating and rehabilitating mentally ill patients in community hospitals, so as to reduce human right violations... has resulted in the criminalization of mentally disordered behavior.*
>
> *Jimmy Carter's commission on mental health greatly articulated the goals but had no agency to accomplish them. The object of marinating the greatest degree of freedom, self determination, autonomy, dignity and integrity of body, mind and spirit for the individual while he or she participates in treatment or receives services, was noble but not doable...*
>
> *For a substantial numbers, Deinstituionalization has become a psychiatric titanic. Their lives are virtually devoid of dignity of mind, body and spirit. Self determination often means merely that the person has a choice of soup kitchens. The least restricted setting frequently turns out to be a cardboard box, a jail cell, or a terror filled existence on the streets."*

And the inhumane treatment of mixing the mentally ill with hardened criminals, as was common a century and a half ago, is proving a lethal mix.

On May 8, 2009, guards at the Wallens Ridge Prison in Virginia found the bound body of 63 year old Harvey Gray who had been, gagged, beaten and then strangled to death by another prisoner, Robert Gleason Jr. The death had gone unnoticed for almost a day before being discovered by authorities.

The two were cell mates. Living together in an 8-by 10- foot cell, Gleason was vexed by Watson's erratic behaviors. He pleaded with prison officials to find him another cell before he snapped. But the request went unheeded and the constant screaming, and obscenity laced tirades, was pushing Gleason over the edge.

When his cry for help continued to go unheeded, Gleason took matters into his own hands.

Gleason used slivers of bed sheets to tie Watson's hands and arms to his body. He fashioned a gag out of two pillow cases which he later removed to give Watson a cigarette. When Watson spit the cigarette back in his face, Gleason jumped on his cellmate, beat him, and strangled him to death.

He then covered Watson's body with a bed sheet to make it look like he was sleeping and was able to keep the murder a secret through two mandatory standing counts and two meals. The discovery was made when Watson's psychiatrist came in to see him and found him dead.

After the closing of Pennsylvania's Allentown State Hospital in January of 2010, a startling statistic was discovered. The number of state prisons had recently climbed from 6 to 27. During the same period, the number of states mental hospitals had declined from 22 to 6. A telling trend. Unfortunately, the trend is national.

An estimated 25-30 % of those now in the state prisons are for crimes committed while being mentally ill.

In perhaps the greatest infringement of human rights in American history, citizens are now being incarcerated without legitimately having committed a crime.

And what about the potential danger posed by the mentally ill who are homeless and wander the streets? One writer commenting on the violence occurring to and by the mentally ill, acknowledged this:

> *"The closing of mental health treatment centers will only lead to future violence in our communities. Without a change in our current polices, future violence is assured. That means that there are future victims waiting to pay the ultimate price for our current policy maker failures." (3)*

One needs only to look at Columbine, the massacre at Virginia Tech University and the Tucson slayings as evidence that the present mental health model is failing everyone.

In the popular Yahoo Forum YaHoo! ANSWERS, there is the following question and answer.

Why did the government close many mental institutions?

Best Answer-Chosen by Voters

"Yes, the excuse for closing them down was it was thought it better for them to live in community housing. In reality the government made a fortune when they sold off the mental institutions (most of them were on prime land) The problem is the mentally ill that were residing in mental institutions were there because they needed supervision, especially when it comes to taking their medication. Without supervision and medication...arguments, bullying and violence developed in the community homes and consequently a lot of them are now living on the streets where they feel safer.

Creating mental institutions would cut our homeless population significantly. Unfortunately the public hospital system is struggling to keep its head above water as it is, so I see no light at the end of the tunnel for the mentally ill."

Φ Φ Φ Φ Φ Φ Φ Φ Φ Φ Φ Φ Φ Φ Φ Φ Φ Φ

UP TO THIS POINT, I had no real experience in seeing first hand the plight of the mentally ill. That all changed quite unexpectedly on Christmas day while visiting friends after Christmas dinner.

On the spur of the moment, I jumped in my car to visit on old friend who had recently moved to a new location in a nearby town. As I entered the living room where his family had gathered, there sat his ex-wife Maggie.

I had not seen Maggie in several years. I remembered her as a bright, beautiful woman, with sparkling eyes and a quick wit. She had completely swept my friend Roger off his feet when they first met. They soon married and began to raise a family.

But things took a turn for the worse after Maggie visited a spiritualist medium. Later she told me that God had visited her one day as she lay on a bed in an upstairs bedroom. A voice said that God wanted to come inside her and that he would make her rich and give her power.

There began a toboggan slide downward in her life. Substance abuse, gambling, and sexual immorality led her to leave her husband and family. Violent outbursts led her to have altercations with the law.

When her ex-husband visited at her apartment one day, he found her disassembling a boom box and the television set looking for voices. He got in touch with mental health services, who recommended he take her to the emergency room.

The next years saw her in and out of court, in and out of emergency rooms, in and out of the lives of her children and ex husband. It was only after her outbursts were considered a threat to the community that she had a stay at Riverview Psychiatric Center, only to be released after about a month.

As I looked across the room and saw her sitting on the couch I could barley believe I was seeing the same person. Those eyes, once so engaging were dim, lifeless, and vacant.

Maggie would listen to our conversations, laugh inappropriately and leave the room. Just as a cancer ravages the human body, this illness had ravaged her mind.

Or maybe it wasn't an illness. Maybe those paranormals and exorcists understand a facet of human existence that our secularized minds are having great difficulty in wrapping around.

With the hour getting late, I volunteered to give Maggie a ride back to her apartment. We had a long, perfectly coherent conversation, recalling people and places from our past.

She asked if we could stop at the store so she could pick up some Christmas gifts for her friends. She directed me to stop at a beverage store where she bought several bottles of hard liquor.

As we turned into the driveway of her apartment complex, it reminded me of a 1950's shanty town. No, it reminded me of the Bates Motel of Psycho fame. Run down and shabby, I shuttered to think what I might find on the inside as I helped with her bags and presents.

As we entered her tiny two room rent, I was bowled over by the smell of decaying food, empty beer cans and a smoldering marijuana joint. Her bed lie un-made in the middle of the room, clothes and trash strewn there and about.

I quickly and politely let myself out of the apartment only to be greeted by Greg, who lived a few doors down. "Could you give my friend Greg a ride to the store to get some supplies for the week?" Maggie asked. I nodded yes.

Greg gave me instructions to go to the same beverage store. He returned to my vehicle with 2 cases of Miller Light and a carton of cigarettes. I dropped him off in front of his room with the request that he take care of Maggie. "Oh yes, of course I will", he responded. "She is coming over right after you leave."

As I drove off, I angrily thought to myself, "Is this the Department of Health and Human Services answer to the problem of treating the mentally ill? If it is, we have come full circle. We are back to before 1840, when sufferers were incarcerated in prisons, jails, and dumps like this."

A few months later I saw Maggie again, this time on the front page of the daily newspaper. She had started a fire in her apartment, nearly killing herself and the 14 others who occupied the building.

The time has come for us to force our elected officials into putting the necessary money and effort into curing and helping the mentally ill rather than the useless endeavors of putting man on the Moon... Or Mars... Or Afghanistan.

APPENDIX

Post mortem evaluation:

She was born Mary Theresa McConnell on March 26th 1929 in Norridgewock, Maine. She was adopted by Silvier F. Sirois and Rose T. Sirois. Consent was given by Madeline Sirois, supposedly the mother. Parents were named as Albert McConnell and Madeline Sirois. At adoption her name was changed to Mary Constance Sirois. At the age of two she and her adopted father went to live with his daughter, Mrs. Warren Marcoux. Mr. Marcoux had two children by a previous marriage. Mrs. Marcoux had in all twelve children, some lost in childbirth and one of whom was crippled. Those who lived a home with the patient were Bobby, Virginia' Jacqueline, Bunny, Louise and Billy. In age, patient was between the two others daughters and people often mistook them for triplets.

EDUCATION

She attended Mount Merici Academy for four years, 1934-1938. She then attended Waterville Maine Public schools for one year. At this her foster mother describe her as difficult to handle and high spirited.

Since the mother was expecting a baby she sent her daughter to the Sacred Heart Academy in Jackman, Maine until 1941. She then attended Mount Merici High School for three years. At school she was not conceded very sociable. Her grades were much below her mental ability. She read constantly. She was considered stubborn and difficult to handle. Her I.Q. was then 133.

MEDICAL

At age eight, she had a T&A. At age ten she had and appendectomy. She began menstruation at age twelve or thirteen.

EMPLOYMENT

After school she was employed as a part time worker as a bakers helper at the Harris Baking Co. in Waterville, Maine. She worked at the 4:00 AM to 8:00 AM shift. She was employed there from Sept. 12, 1945 to June 5, 1946. She was considered dependable and regular in attendance.

MARRIAGE

She was married on June 29, 1946, to Carl Merrill Fisher, nine years older. He was employed by Mine Central Railroad in the car shop. Her husband was devoted to her and their sex life was very satisfactory. They lived with his parents for a short time. They go along well and were very kind to her. They then bought a camp at Snow Pond which consisted of a cedar log cabin of two rooms without running water or indoor toilet. Water had to be hauled from a spring one hundred feet away. She had to get wash water from the lake because the water from the spring was too hard. In the winter, they had to chop through three or four feet of ice. The had an oil stove and had two fires scare and switched to coal but she worried about the coal gas.

PERSONALITY

One of her sisters described her as a young girl who was gay, high spirited always in hot water, a leader of the gang of children. The sister
stated that after marriage, the patient became a quiet person who never
complained and never talked about anything. In later interviews the
patients husband stated her family had made fun of her because she
wanted to be clean and shampooed her hair frequently. He said Constance, (who was called Peggy by the family,) was much better looking
than the others kids. He also said she was smarter and had more boy-
friends and implied they were all jealous of her. The patient stated in
hospital interviews that she felt rejected by the family at being sent away
to school and also that they had sent her back to school while she was
still ill. Her husband described her as quick tempered but would never
hold a grudge. She would fly off the handle at little things. She loved
to cook and collect recipes. She enjoyed reading and loved to write poetry. She was friendly but had no close friends, she enjoyed needlework
and handiwork of all kinds.

PREGANANCIES

She had been married for only a week when she became pregnant for
the first time. After three unplanned children, she decided not to have
any more children, so her husband used prophylactics. In later interviews, she claimed not to know that the Catholic Church was against
birth control. When she later found out, she felt guilty but had to use
it because she didn't want another baby.

She was attended by Dr. Sam Fisher through all three pregnancies
at the Seton Hospital in Waterville, Maine. They were all normal and
uneventful. She nursed the last baby.

ONSET OF ILLNESS

In November 1953, after weaning the baby, she began having sudden spells of depression which were worse just before and during her menstrual periods. She also suffered chronic sinitis and ear infections. The depression spells became worse after Christmas and one day she tried to strangle the baby with a scarf but it woke up and made a sound and she stopped. Once she took her fathers gun to kill them all but then took the gun back, twice again she did the same thing.

After she had lost a great deal of weight and continued to feel depressed and confused, her husband took her to see Dr. R.L. Chasse, M.D. of Waterville, Maine. He had treated her for anemia in pregnancy in July, 1954. He saw her on January 21, 1954. She complained of insomnia, nervousness and feeling run down. Dr. Chasse recommended then that they over into town, away from their isolated little cottage where they lived away from other families. He prescribed Phenobarbital after meals and at bedtime. He saw her again on February 4, 1954. She was dramatically improved was eating well sleeping well going out shipping etc. Dr. Chasse did a CBC found anemia and prescribed oral iron, IM injections of folic acid B12 and an antigenic diet. She got one injection of February 25, but did not comeback for more. Around February 11, 1954 Dr. Chasse was called to her home by Dr. Sam Fisher, her gynecologist after she had take an overdose of Phenobarbital which was thought to be accidental. Dr. Chasse recommend that she see Dr. Stebbins of Bangor. But they preferred to consult Dr. Paul Jones of Union, Maine who had been recommended by Dr. Fisher.

PSYCHIATRIC TREATMENT

By now the Fishers had move into an apartment in Waterville with four rooms and a bath.

On February 14, 1954 Dr. Paul Jones saw her in his office in Union, Maine. There was a mix-up in time and transportation and he could only see her for only twenty minutes. His initial diagnosis was mild depression, possibly situational and informed her parents that the patient was a potential suicide and recommend close observation until a more extensive study could be done in Waterville at the Mansfield Clinic.

On February 23, 1954 Dr. Jones saw her again at the Mansfield Clinic for an hour. She denied any feelings of depression and claimed to be feeling fine and having no trouble eating or sleeping. She was very cheerful during the interview. Dr. Jones felt the patient had had a situation depression which had been corrected by moving to town. Later in the day her foster mother phoned to say she had found a noted from the patient that indicated the patient might destroy herself. This surprised Dr. Jones, being a such variance with his observations. He advised Mrs. Marcoux to keep a close watch on her for other symptoms and unusual behavior.

FIRST SET OF MURDERS

On March 8, 1954 Carl Fisher arrived home after work to find all three children drowned. The older boy was face down in the bathtub and the younger boy and girl were in their beds covered with blankets. His wife was lying under the bed, semi- conscious with a partially empty bottle of Selsum Shampoo beside her.

Dr. Chasse was called in and the patient said to him " Thy are safe in heaven now, where I want them to be. The only mistake I made is not being successful in killing myself."

Mrs. Fisher left a lengthy note written of a paper bag, begging her husbands forgiveness an saying that she loved them all very much. She expressed hope that they would all be together again someday.

FIRST HOSPITALIZATION

Mrs. Fisher was admitted to the Augusta State Hospital under a Superior Court Commitment. The original diagnosis was Schizophrenia, Paranoid Type. Her physical exam showed her to be in good health except anemic. An EEG showed no abnormal features. A psychologist report done n March 17, 1954 stated patient was cheerful, showed no sign of grief, sorrow or anxiety. She smile frequently and had an innocent and childlike manner. Her IQ was 125. She expressed a wish to have more children.

During an interview with Dr. Sleeper and Dr. Marquardt on May 25, 1954 she said she had been worried about money. She heard voices in her mind, didn't know if it was God or not, couldn't decide. She smiled when she said she felt awful about killing the children. She said it was if someone else took control of her. She prayed to God to tell her what to do. She became calm, it seemed as if she were an onlooker, looking at a movie.

After period of observation, she was she was given insulin shock therapy. Staff observed her having auditory hallucinations.

Her husband and her family were very devoted an supportive of her, visiting frequently and bring her food, gifts and material for handiwork.

After several petitions for release she was granted a request for discharge on May 6, 1959.

STARTING OVER

While his wife had been in the hospital, Mr. Fisher had saved his money and purchased a farm in Fairfield, Maine. It consisted of a house with four rooms and a bath downstairs, two unfinished rooms upstairs, a barn and 70 acres of land. Mr. George Greeley, a social worker visited Mr. Fisher at the farm five days and again two days before Mrs. Fisher's discharge He found Mr. Fisher laid off from work, depressed and apathetic. He found the house somewhat depressing.

Subsequently, Mrs Fisher bore three more children, two girls and a boy. She was attended at each birth by Dr. Edgar Smith of Fairfield at Seton Hospital. Dr. Price Kirkpatrick saw her after each of the births. He found he to be free of any psychotic symptoms.

Her sister stated her own children were very fond of their aunt and uncle. The Fisher farm was an ideal place for children with goats and kittens. The Fisher children had every possible toy, expensive books, records doll for the girl and a tractor for the boy. Mrs. Fisher nursed all three children.

In March 1966, a priest suggested that Mrs. Fisher was very depressed and not doing any housework and Dr. Kirkpatrick started on a drug program of Prolixin and Tofranil and Placidyl for sleep. He was seen again in June on emergency. She had stopped medication. She was admitted to Seton Hospital. She was given Mellaril and Nardil. While in the hospital she was visited often by her husband and she taped recorded messages for the children. She was discharged after five days. Dr. Kirkpatrick later said mistakenly diagnosed her condition as Postpartum Psychosis, Depressive Reactions.

SECOND SET OF MURDERS

After her release from the hospital, Mr. Fisher had taken a few days off from work to help his wife around the house. The day he went back to work, as soon as he had left the house, Mrs. Fisher again drowned the children. In the same manner as the first, the older child was face down in the bath tub and the younger children were left in their beds. Mrs. Fisher again tried to kill herself by taking an overdose of sleeping pills.

SECOND ADMISSION

Mrs. Fisher was again admitted to ASH on July 6, 1966 on Superior Court Commitment. While in the hospital, patient had auditory hallucinations and suffered from religious delusions. As a patient, she was very cooperative about work and taking own medication. She started behavior modification treatment. She went though job training and a report stated she achieved maximum benefits. There were several petitions for release but her doctors testified against it and they were denied.

Her husband refused to have any more sexual relations with her and eventually refused to see her. A boarding classification was sought but the patient didn't want to live in a boarding home. The husband was adamant about not taking her home. She became overweight again. Around this time, she stated she would like more children.

CASE CLOSED

At 8:PM on October 1, 1973 she was found missing from the ward. Her body as found in the Kennebec River on October 6, 1973. She had drowned.

Notes from the investigation afterwards state that the staff had felt hopeless with the patient and felt there would be no further improvement. Active psychotherapy might have helped staff to be more interested in possibility of effective change. It appears to have been a hospital sanctioned suicide when all hope of improvement in living conditions were closed following the Supreme Court hearing. She was deprived of a place to live for rest of her life.

THE DEAD CHILDREN

First Set: **Richard, 6   Daniel, 4   Deborah, 11 months.**

Second Set: **Kathleen Louise, 6   Michael Jon, 4
Natalie Rose, 9 months.**

REFERENCE NOTES

Chapter One

1) All hospital interviews, police reports, test results and medical evaluations are taken from Mrs. Fisher's medical files.
2) Detailed accounts of the first Fisher murders are contained in the February 9,10, editions of the Bangor Daily News and the Waterville Sentinel.

Chapter Two

1) Sagadahock country probate court record concerning the adoption of Mary Theresa McConnell.
2) Shortly after Maine had achieved statehood in 1820, a statute was provided by the Maine legislature for a type of insanity defense. The statue was revised in 1954, to include the treatment and release of forensic patients.

Chapter Three

1) Maslow's hierarchy of needs is universally recognized as a standard in judging the quality of human life. It ranges from the basics of food and shelter all the way to complete personal fulfillment which he called self actualization.
2) Year end hospital reports for the Maine Insane Hospital are catalogued at the Maine State Library. They continue almost without interruption through 2004 when AMHI was closed by the state legislature.
3) 1st Samuel 21:13-15 is the story of king David feigning madness before king Achish.
4) The message Dorothea Dix presented before the Massachusetts legislature was actually read by another, as women were not allowed to speak before the assembly.

Chapter Four

1) An excerpt from "**The Kennedy Women, by Lawrence Leamer**, (as it appeared on the web site Fat Boy.cc) For all her trouble Rosemary inspired her brother, President John F. Kennedy to promote awareness and later legislation aid to those suffering with mental infirmities.
2) Sakel's experiments were later criticized and repudiated by medical authorities. They called Insulin shock therapy unscientific and inhumane and by the 1970's the procedure and was barred in most states.
3) The eulogy excerpt is taken from a catholic website and titled "**Eulogy for a Baby who dies after Baptism.**" While intended to bring comfort to grieving families, it may have provided Mrs. Fisher the motivation she needed to kill her children.
4) Matthew 18:5,6

Chapter Five

1) Before his death in 2003, Derek Prince was considered to be a leading authority on demons and their operation. His most comprehensive work on the subject is titled, **"They shall expel demons, what you need to know abut demons-your invisible enemies."**
2) Much of the teaching and ministry of Christ involved exposing and expelling demonic spirits. This account is taken from Luke 8:26-39.

CHAPTER SEVEN

1) All names followed by an asterisk are fictitious.

Chapter Eight

1) The interviews were done in person. In so doing, the writer could gauge the emotion in which a response was given. While there was obvious sympathy for Mrs. Fisher, the crimes she committee were considered off the chart deplorable by those interviewed.
2) Information from Dr. Resnick was acquired via telephone and a lecture supplement from his class on filicide.

Chapter Nine

1) The quote from doctor Ray is taken from his 1842, superintendents report of the Maine Insane Hospital. It is of interest that the state of Maine produced two of the leading figures in the mental health reform movement of the 19ᵗʰ century, Dorothea Dix and Dr. Isaac Ray. Quotations in this chapter are taken from his year end reports of 1841-45.
2) An excerpt from Ingersol's book titled **"Crimes against Criminals.**

Interestingly, Vladimir Lenin used the template of Ingersol's argument to blame capitalism for criminality in the west.

Chapter Ten

1) Journalist Brooks Hamilton was one of three reporters to whom Dr. Sleeper granted special access. His report was written in 1949, for the Daily Kennebec Journal, followed by articles done by Peter Damborg of the Portland Sunday Telegram, in 1955, and Ed Kisonak in 1957, for the Lewiston Journal.

Chapter Eleven

1) The eugenics movement led to the establishment of industrial school for girls across the nation such as the one in Hallowell, that had as it goal not only to keep those mentally disabled or delinquent from the rest of society, but also to make sure they would not "sire more of their kind."

Chapter Fourteen

1) The quotation is from the October 11, 1973 edition of the Kennebec Journal. Senator Hichens would continue to hold a fire under administrators and legislators, declaring a probe not only for the Fisher suicide but also the deinstituionalization movement in general. Unfortunately, he did not stay in office long enough to complete them.

Chapter Sixteen

1) An excerpt from a speech by president Kennedy titled **"The Dream."**
2) Quote taken from an article titled **"Mental Health clinics closing-Guaranteeing future violence."** Chicago justice. Org.

ABOUT THE AUTHOR

Bob Briggs is a freelance writer, born and raised in Maine.

He is the author of four books, two about his hometown of Hallowell, and two on the University of Maine where he earned a Bachelors of Arts Degree in History in 1980.

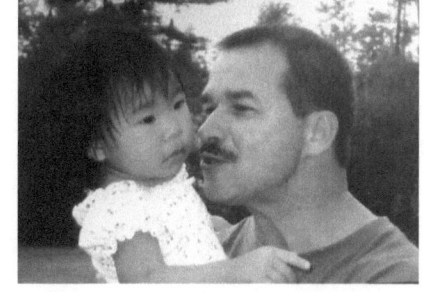

Briggs has worked as a reporter for the Kennebec Journal and The Capitol Weekly. He was a religion writer for 10 years.

He is a certified school teacher, and taught four years in public schools. He has served on the board of directors for Grace Christian Academy in West Gardiner, Maine. He is an advocate for making child safety a national priority.

www.ingramcontent.com/pod-product-compliance
Lightning Source LLC
Chambersburg PA
CBHW030254290526
45785CB00001B/81